# YOUR BODY
# HIS TEMPLE

# YOUR BODY
# HIS TEMPLE

## Dr. Alfred L. Heller

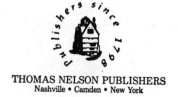

THOMAS NELSON PUBLISHERS
Nashville • Camden • New York

Third printing

Published in Nashville, Tennessee, by Thomas Nelson, Inc. and distributed in Canada by Lawson Falle, Ltd., Cambridge, Ontario.

Printed in the United States of America.

Scripture quotations are from the New American Standard Bible, © The Lockman Foundation 1960, 1962, 1963, 1968, 1971, 1972, 1973, 1975, and are used by permission.

Drawings in Chapter 7 by Rose Teasley.

Library of Congress Cataloging in Publication Data

Heller, Alfred L.
  Your body, his temple.

  Bibliography: p. 190
  1. Health.   2. Exercise.   3. Diet.   4. Christian life—1960–
I. Title.

RA776.5.H4          613.2          81–1897
ISBN 0–8407–5769–7          AACR2

This book is dedicated
to my wife,
Wanda,
and our children,
Kerry, Rob, and Jenny,
who encouraged me
when most needed.

# Acknowledgments

The following people were very helpful in their suggestions, manuscript editing, and willingness to help this book to become a reality: Dr. Richard O'Brien, Dr. Donald Furci, Dr. Roger Hirchak, Tom Bernard (my running partner), Jan Bernard (who contributed material for the discussion on sugar), Conrad Carnes, Tom Driskell, Pastor Jim Custer, Pastor Dick Mayhue, Pastor John Willett, and my best friend and wife, Wanda (who contributed material for Chapter 12). Thanks also to Evelyn Barkman for editing and typing the original manuscript and to Sharon Waller for typing the final manuscript.

# Contents

# List of Tables

# Foreword

Even though man has been on earth for many thousands of years, he knows very little about how his body works. Unvarnished facts stagger the imagination. Sixty trillion cells function in a typical middle-aged American man. Each one is a microscopic city with power stations, a transportation system, a communications network. Raw materials are manufactured and waste is disposed. Each cell operates efficiently and polices itself to keep out undesirables.

This remarkable mechanism is nourished by a splendidly rich 75,000-mile bloodstream, and is presided over by a three-pound gray and white mushroom, a brain of 30 billion neurons, the myriad functions of which have never been even remotely duplicated.

When I as a person understand that I am made in the image of God, that I am so infinitely precious to the Creator that Jesus Christ died to save me, and that God wants to show Himself through my body, then it matters very much how I treat this miracle of flesh and blood I have been given.

*Your Body, His Temple* comes from the pen of a medically knowledgeable doctor who cares most about the ultimate use of the body for its highest purposes, both physically and spiritually.

Dr. Heller glimpses the glory of the assignment humans have in caring for their bodies. He has treated a neglected, and often avoided, subject. Our world is hard on humanity; our life-styles decimate satisfying and effective living. In recent years chunks of undigested medical information have been dumped into the mass media. Not knowing what to believe, many of us ignore basic health rules.

Diets, exercise, additives, and attitudes are skillfully explained. The reader is led through a series of ideas into a logical and God-honoring conclusion about himself. A contract with the Creator is included. If we are serious about honoring the lease of three-score and ten on our personal physical property, we need to read—and to practice—what this book tells us.

Howard G. Hendricks
Professor of Christian Education
Dallas Theological Seminary

# CHAPTER 1

## Understanding Ourselves

This book is written to help you better understand your body. I will address the physical makeup of the body; how food is turned into energy; how to exercise properly; the importance of high calorie foods; and what the Bible tells us about taking care of our bodies.

Our bodies really are something *special*. We were created in the image of God, and that is reason enough to learn how to take care of the bodies that God has entrusted to us.

A balanced diet and good health are relatively easy to obtain, especially if we look to the Lord for motivation and guidance. Every human being cares what he or she looks like and what other people think of him or her. We all would like to be healthy and to know how to determine our ultimate health by the food we eat.

Exercise should be understood so that we don't avoid it because of false information. This book gives the basic underlying truth about exercise, how to obtain health through exercise, and what exercise to use in maintaining a healthy body.

You may ask—and quite legitimately—why a book is needed to speak to personal health care from a Christian standpoint. Isn't that something like producing a *Christian Auto Repair Manual* or a *Believers' Guide for Lawn and Garden?* Not at all. Remember: A Christian is in personal union with Jesus Christ. Our bodies are temples of the Holy Spirit. So, in contrast to a car or a tulip bulb, we enjoy a unique relationship with God, as His property.

But there are other differences, too. The way a person with a biblical orientation views himself will (or at least, *should*) be far higher than the manner in which a secular person sees himself. When we understand God's viewpoint of our redeemed humanity, our self-image soars! Further, a Christian's motivation for the care and maintenance of the human frame is different from that of one who is not in touch with Jesus Christ. Paul said, "I can do all things through Him who strengthens me" (Phil. 4:13). The natural man may have the *desire* to stay fit; the Christian has the *power* to stay fit.

Yes, there are incredible differences in the way a child of God can be challenged and instructed to care for himself. If you are in Christ, your ability to hear from God and to know His will, your motivation for righteousness and health, and your God-given power and determination to obey the truth is, *by His promise*, far superior to those outside His covenant. So, Christian, take heart! The Enabler will stand with you in dealing with yourself.

## What Got Me Going

I have always been interested in physical activity and eating nutritious food, but it wasn't until God impressed on me the need to share my ideas and experiences that this book became a reality.

I suppose all of us need some sort of jolt—mild or major—to startle us out of complacency to start us taking care of ourselves. Since my experience is representative of that of many men over thirty, permit me to tell you my own story.

While in high school I participated in football, basketball, track, and baseball. I lifted weights for strength and ran in the off-season to stay in shape. Playing football as a senior, I weighed 162 pounds, was five feet nine inches tall, and ate everything in sight to keep that weight. I remember eating three large meals a day plus three snacks—one at night before going to bed included one-half gallon of chocolate ice cream and a full bag of potato chips.

During the summer months I was a lifeguard and can remember my mother daily bringing me milkshakes containing eggs, protein supplements, and a half-gallon of ice cream. I drank these just trying to keep weight on my frame for football. As you know, a growing boy needs to eat!

From 17 to 25 I played college soccer and lacrosse. In dental college my exercise program consisted of playing basketball at lunchtime for one-and-a-half hours. During this period my weight stayed at 162 pounds. At age 25 I entered the military and found my time for athletics was limited to softball and golf. At age 28 I left the service and started private dental practice. My weight was still 162, even though I was eating like a pig three meals a day and getting very little exercise. I usually had only one snack per day.

After being in dental practice for two years and working many long, strenuous hours, I celebrated my thirtieth birthday at 162 pounds. I remember telling my wife that it must be my hard work and the fact that I was coaching little league football and baseball that allowed me to keep my high school weight.

From age 30 to 33 I gained 21 pounds, even though I was watching what I ate more closely. After all, I was a doctor. Didn't I know what not to eat to avoid getting fat?

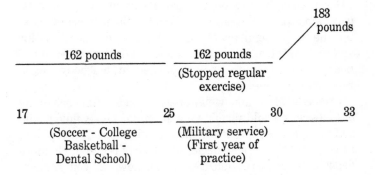

## Subtle Degeneration

*Let's clarify this!* I stopped regular exercise at age 25; yet my weight remained constant until I was 30. Did I diet? The answer is definitely no. I ate whatever I wished. The only thing I did differently was to cut my snacks and stop regular exercise. From age 30 to 33, why did I gain 21 pounds if my diet was the same as in the previous five years? The answer is quite simple. My muscles were slowly being infiltrated with fatty tissue. It is such a slow process, my body took *five years* before the scale showed the difference.

When we are active and exercise on a regular basis, such as playing high school sports, our muscles are efficient machines. The foods we eat (carbohydrates, proteins, and fats) are metabolized to keep that machine running efficiently. When I stopped exercising at age 25, my muscles were still efficient machines. From age 25 to 30, due to lack of exercise my machine became less effective, but it weighed the same 162 pounds.

If a muscle is not exercised, it will atrophy (shrink up) in size. As an example, if you have ever had your leg in a cast for six weeks, you will remember the sick feeling when the cast was removed and you first looked at your atrophied muscle. The leg was less than one-half the size of the other healthy leg.

Even though we stop exercising our muscles, our diets usually consist of the same food intake. When muscle shrinks up, the body chemistry changes and fat is deposited within and around the atrophied muscle cell. With the retention of body fluid added to this new deposited fat, our body weight remains the same.

I remained the same weight because every time one of my muscles cells would shrink, fat and retained body fluid would add up to the weight of the muscle cell before it atrophied. Finally, at 30, my body declared, "End of the line. No more depositing fat in the muscles. From now on, you glutton, *excess fat will be deposited outside of the muscle.*"

This is called *subcutaneous fat,* otherwise known as spare tires, love handles, and flabby cheeks.

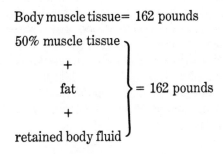

Body muscle tissue= 162 pounds

50% muscle tissue

\+

fat                          = 162 pounds

\+

retained body fluid

From age 30 to 33 I continued to eat and my body continued to deposit the excess calories as subcutaneous fat. An interesting fact should be noted: During this three-year period, I actually ate less because I was very busy building a dental practice, and I was gradually becoming embarrassed with my physical appearance. I would go several days eating only one meal and then take my wife out to eat Friday evening to make up for depriving myself. It was shocking for me to eat one or two small meals per day Monday through Thursday and then, after eating what I wanted on Friday evening, to find Saturday morning that our bathroom scale claimed I was one pound heavier. I asked myself, "Why?"

I tried lots of different diets and many types of diet pills. The diets worked for a short period of time, but then the darn old bathroom scale would show me the truth. New scales did not make any difference. I was a fat glob! *A foodaholic!*

### What About You?

Stop and think about your own body. Did you experience a similar subtle time schedule in becoming out of shape or overweight? Think about your past struggles with weight. Is there a similar chain of events? Most people answer yes. Dr. Richard O'Brien, a good friend who works very hard to stay in shape, calls this phenomenon "creeping obesity."

In health surveys, when adults are asked to choose between success, love, sex, fame, fortune, or good health, do you know what they select? Good health *always* tops the list as the most desired possession.

Dr. Donald Furci, a Christian physician and friend, has a simple, helpful classification for his patients which shows that human life is made up of four basic components. Personal happiness seems to be the highest when these elements are in balance:

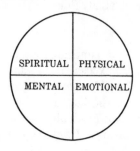

1 Thess. 5:23:
" . . . may your spirit and soul and body be preserved complete. . . ."

If any one of these segments is out of proportion, the other three suffer. If we are involved only with spiritual things every waking moment, it becomes obvious that other areas of our life are out of balance, especially if we are expected to be the head of a household. If we are not emotionally rested and stable when facing a crisis, our spiritual, mental, and physical segments will not be able to function at the level they should for good balance.

Similarly, Dr. L. D. Panky, a dental colleague, has used a

"cross of life" illustration to show that work, play, love, and worship should be kept in balance in order to have a happy and full life. If we work too much, we won't have time for worship, play, or personal relationships.

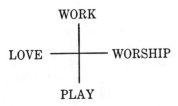

This book emphasizes how to keep the physical aspect of our lives in balance. Proverbs 1:7 tells us, ". . . Fools despise wisdom and instruction." Do you know what God expects from us concerning our physical appearance? Our eating habits? Does God want us to exercise? Does God care if we are fat? Let's go first to His Word to find His instructions.

# CHAPTER 2

## Borrowed Property

The Scriptures tell us in no uncertain terms that God cares about our health.

The apostle Paul tells us, "Do you not know that you are a temple of God, and that the Spirit of God dwells in you? If any man destroys the temple of God, God will destroy him, for the temple of God is holy, and that is what you are" (1 Cor. 3:16,17).

In these verses, God reveals that each of us is an individual temple which houses His Spirit. We have a choice to either destroy or maintain a healthy temple. God leaves no lingering doubt about His will for His temple. If a person destroys that temple, *God will destroy him.* This is serious business.

He continues, "Do you not know that your body is a temple of the Holy Spirit who is in you, whom you have from God, and that you are not your own? For you have been bought with a price: therefore glorify God in your body" (1 Cor. 6:19,20).

If you were to borrow your father's brand new car for a special reason, would you take care of it? You probably would be more careful with a borrowed automobile than with a car you owned. As I understand the verses in 1 Corinthians, our bodies are on loan to us. They are borrowed in the sense that they are the property of someone else. We were bought with a price, the sacrifice of Jesus Christ. Thus, we are instructed to glorify God through our bodies. Are you proud of your body? Do you take care of it?

Elsewhere in his writings, Paul teaches, "For many walk,

of whom I often told you, and now tell you even weeping, that they are enemies of the cross of Christ, whose end is destruction, whose god is their appetite, and whose glory is in their shame, who set their minds on earthly things" (Phil. 3:18,19).

And in that familiar word to Rome: "Now I urge you, brethren, keep your eyes on those who cause dissensions and hindrances contrary to the teaching which you learned, and turn away from them. For such men are slaves, not of our Lord Christ but of their own *appetites;* and by their smooth and flattering speech they deceive the hearts of the unsuspecting" (Rom. 16:17,18; italics mine).

## Why Do We Eat?

Do you eat to live or do you live to eat? Do you put down the knife and fork from breakfast and ask, "What's for lunch?" The Bible tells us that our appetite drives must be controlled. These drives include sleep, sex, food, or other areas of our lives that when misused keep us from being a healthy temple of God.

Do you ever get the feeling that we Americans view gluttony, alcoholic consumption, reckless driving, sexual frenzy, and smoking as constitutional rights? Dr. Thomas Bassler, a pathologist, tells us that on the basis of the many autopsies he has performed, *two out of every three deaths are premature.* He believes these deaths are the result of "smoker's lung," "loafer's heart," and "drinker's liver." (10)* Smoker's lung is a result of the daily pollution of lungs with cigarettes. Loafer's heart is a result of spending more time in front of the TV set than walking. Drinker's liver is a result of polluting that organ with alcohol until it is incapable of fighting disease.

---

*Numbers appearing in parentheses in the text refer to the entry (or entries) in the bibliography from which quoted or background material was obtained.

Thomas K. Cureton, of the University of Illinois Physical Fitness Laboratory, has said, "The average American young man has a middle-aged body. He can't run the length of a city block; he can't climb a flight of stairs without getting breathless." (24)

James F. Fixx, in his book *The Complete Book of Running*, states that "fifty million adult Americans never exercise, and even American *kids* are out of shape." He cites a study showing that in one Massachusetts school only eight fifth-graders out of a class of 52 were fit enough to earn the President's Physical Fitness Award. In a class in Connecticut, only two students out of forty qualified. Fixx also alluded to a study at Massachusetts General Hospital which showed that 15 percent of nineteen hundred seventh-graders had high cholesterol levels and eight percent had high blood pressure. (24) (Both conditions are risk factors which increase the chances of a heart attack.)

## Fit for His Service

Without wanting to press the issue too far, there are some intriguing situations in the Scriptures that show that our forebearers in the faith were, by and large, people who were in shape. For openers, it would be safe to assume that God did not create Adam fat! On the other hand, many of the pagan kings were fat, and probably considered it an honor. Let's look at some of the saints and prophets of the Old and New Testaments.

Genesis 37:13–17 tells us that Joseph had to *walk* 50 miles to get to his brothers, and he was only a teen-ager at the time.

Exodus 5:17–19 tells us God brought circumstances to the Hebrews held captive in Egypt that caused them to work hard physically for long hours. This effort required that they be (or perhaps *caused* them to be) in good physical shape to survive. Being in good physical condition, they were prepared for the long and strenuous *walk* into the Promised Land.

Deuteronomy 34:1 tells us that Moses, God's chosen man to lead the Jews out of captivity, was still able to *climb* Pisgah Peak in Mount Nebo at the age of 120 years. Don't forget that Moses, being a leader, probably *walked* ahead of his flock on many occasions. It is safe to believe that Moses was always fit while serving the Lord, for Deuteronomy 34:7 tells us that "although Moses was one hundred and twenty years old when he died, his eye was not dim, nor his vigor [energy] abated." How else could he have had vigor at age 120?

Joshua 6:3 states, "And you shall *march* around the city, all the men of war circling the city once. You shall do so for six days" (italics mine). So the sons of Israel were ordered by Joshua to march for six days. Logic tells us that marching would be more strenuous than walking.

Joshua 20:1–9 includes instructions from the Lord to Joshua concerning innocent persons who were *fleeing* for their lives to a designated city of refuge. I can only assume that a person fleeing would be moving out at a fair rate of speed, especially if the avenger of blood was pursuing him.

First Kings 18:46 and 19:1–5 tell us that Elijah *ran* about 20 miles, then fled another 90 miles as he *ran* (19:3) for his life. He then left his servant and ran for a day into the wilderness. At the end of the day he sat down under a juniper tree and fell asleep. How many of us would be fit enough to follow Elijah in his escape?

Mark 6:33 says people *ran* around the Sea of Galilee from all the surrounding cities to get closer to Jesus, who on this occasion was preaching from a boat.

Matthew 15:21 tells us that Jesus *walked* to the districts of Tyre and Sidon, which were some 50 miles away. John 21:7,8 says Peter *swam* about 100 yards to Jesus standing on the shore.

John 20:1,2 shows that Mary Magdalene went to the tomb while it was still dark. Seeing the stone had already been taken away, she *ran* to Jerusalem to tell Peter and John (a trip of approximately three miles). John and Peter ran back to the site of the tomb (20:3) and John (was he in better physical condition?) *ran* faster than Peter (20:4) and reached the vacant tomb first.

Luke 24:13–24 tells of two disciples, one of whom was named Cleopas, who lived in Emmaus. They *walked* from Jerusalem to Emmaus, ate supper, and hurried back to Jerusalem, which was a round trip of about fifteen miles. That is quite a long distance to travel for supper. They must have walked quite briskly, because it was late afternoon before they left Jerusalem.

First Corinthians 9:27 tells us that Paul *buffeted* (disciplined) his body so as not to be disqualified.

Interesting, isn't it? While we would be hard-pressed to build a "theology of running" on these passages, they do, nonetheless, suggest the saints were in shape.

## The Wonder of Our Temple of Clay

David tells us in Psalm 139:13–16:

> For Thou didst form my inward parts;
> Thou didst weave me in my mother's womb.
> I will give thanks to Thee, for I am fearfully and
>   wonderfully made;
> Wonderful are Thy works,
> And my soul knows it very well.
> My frame was not hidden from Thee,
> When I was made in secret,
> And skillfully wrought in the depths of the earth.
> Thine eyes have seen my unformed substance;
> And in Thy book they were all written,
> The days that were ordained for me,
> When as yet there was not one of them.

This passage of Scripture is wonderfully written by David to help us understand how important our bodies really are when viewed by God.

Everything you are had its origin in your mother's womb. Your body and soul were fashioned and woven together according to the foreknowledge and wisdom of God. You were anticipated by His plan before you were conceived. Your conception was ordered by Him to fulfill His plan. That plan included the guidelines for the development of your substance, as the embryo unfolded through all the mysterious processes and became mind and muscle, tissue and thought.

Nothing was added to your being from outside that "unformed substance" as it took its appointed form, i.e., your veins, muscles, inner organs, and your "frame." God interwove your soul and body into one unit. Both your spiritual and physical characteristics were formed and interlocked in your mother's womb.

You are in a state of being as a result of the *sum total* of elements that were made in secret. You are the product of what God made in the dark, mysterious laboratory of the womb, through processes that are beyond our comprehension.

As with Adam, God had an individual plan for you before you were an embryo. You were "skillfully wrought," to be what God wanted you to become. You are no accident, as seen through the eyes of God. All of your potential was present in the embryo, waiting for development through time.

God already saw you as a mature being and already planned for your fulfillment of His plan. In His book He had all your days written, even before any of those days had come to pass.

Are you *physically* what God planned for you to be? Are you *spiritually* what God planned for you to be? We need to restore the value and sacred respect we have lost for our bodies.

Our bodies are wonderful vessels fit for the indwelling of His Majesty, the God of eternity. God needed to visit our human race to redeem us. He still lives in us today. What higher recommendation could be given our "temple of clay"?

### Family Resemblances

One reason God cares so much about us is that we were made in His image. During the act of Creation, the triune God declared, " 'Let Us make man in Our image, according to Our likeness; and let them rule over the fish of the sea and over the birds of the sky and over the cattle and over all the earth, and over every creeping thing that creeps on the earth' " (Gen. 1:26).

We are so worthwhile to Him that even though we fell away from Him through our sins, God the Father sent His eternal Son, by the Holy Spirit in the virgin Mary, to bring us back into His family. Perhaps the best-known verse in all the Bible tells us why. "For God so loved the world, that He gave His only begotten Son, that whoever believes in Him should not perish, but have eternal life" (John 3:16).

You see, if God believes we are worthwhile enough for Him to a) create in the first place, b) make us in His image, and c) come after when we strayed through sin, then we are mighty precious in His sight. From His revelation, we see we are worthwhile in the highest sense of the word. We must guard His investment in us.

Politicians wisely say, "There is nothing more precious to any of us than our health." So we allow them to spend billions on expanded government health programs. In 1977 the nation's health bill rose $14 billion to $118.5 billion, 8.3 percent of the gross national product!

It appears irrational for Americans to spend so much

money to cope with illness, when so much of the illness is the predictable result of poor diet and exercise habits. We are paying increasing sums of private and public money for medicine that treats the consequences of dumb behavior after the fact.

Government is *not* gifted in behavior modification. Politicians *cannot* legislate enough money to get the American people to change their eating habits. Politicians have an incentive to define the health problem as the problem of paying for involuntary illness. But much illness is voluntary in the sense that it afflicts people who possess ample information but refuse to change their behavioral patterns.

As the book of Genesis shows, sin entered the world through a desire to disobey God in the area of food. Taking care of ourselves in what we eat and drink and how we behave is part of our visible role in restoring the marred image of God in us.

With that in mind, I want to lay some factual, even scientific, foundations for you in the next few chapters. But first, I'm asking you to promise me something—that you'll pay close attention.

Often when a writer lays down hard facts, the tendency is for the reader to slip by them to reach the more lively or compelling sections of the book. (I know, because I tend to do this too.) Let me request that you stay alert through this more clinical section of the book so that when I call for action a bit later on, you will know precisely *what* to do and *why*.

# CHAPTER 3

## The Honest-to-Goodness Facts About Disease in the USA

The number one health problem in the United States is heart and blood vessel disease. In 1977, 984,972 people died from diseases of the cardiovascular system, accounting for *52 percent of all deaths*. In 1977 it was estimated that the American people paid $120 billion for all types of health care; a large amount of it was for heart and blood vessel disease. (3) In 1980, Americans were expected to spend $229 billion on health care. In 1979, $1 out of $11 went for health care. (64)

Dr. Ken Cooper, author of *The Aerobics Way*, relayed the following information at a recent workshop: In 1950 the cost of health care in the United States was $12 billion; in 1978 it was $180 billion. In 1950 the cost for an average hospital stay was $167; in 1978 it was $2,140. In 1950 daily hospital costs were $15; in 1978 it was $400. (20)

It is obvious that the way to reduce medical care costs is through *prevention*, not more physicians treating the already sick. For instance, physicians have told us for years that heart disease can be controlled by proper diet, exercise programs, weight maintenance, and eliminating the use of tobacco and alcohol.

During the year 1980, the American Heart Association estimates that 40,810,000 Americans will have some major form of heart or blood vessel disease. (3) Hypertension (high blood pressure) will afflict 34,290,000 (one in four adults); coronary heart disease, 4,240,000; rheumatic heart disease, 1,850,000; and stroke, 1,820,000.

Heart attack was the cause of 729,510 deaths in 1978. There are 4,240,000 people alive today (1980) in the United States who have a history of heart attacks or angina pectoris. Of these people, 350,000 will die of a heart attack before they reach a hospital. (The average victim waits three hours before deciding to seek help.) About 1,500,000 Americans will have a heart attack in 1980 and about 650,000 of them will die.

It takes about three years to compile accurate statistics on deaths in this country. Therefore the latest available figures are from 1978, as tabulated by the American Heart Association.

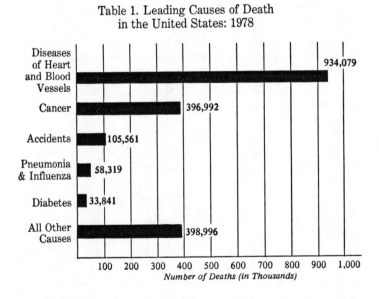

Table 1. Leading Causes of Death
in the United States: 1978

Adapted from National Center for Health Statistics, U.S. Public Health Service DHEW.

## The Big Killers

If you have ever wondered what are the greatest threats to your life you can find out by studying the death rates. There is nothing quite so final as death itself. It is the ultimate statistic. However, the same diseases that cause death can also cause a great deal of suffering. It is a mistake to think that you have a choice between being well and happy or being dead. The quality of life in between varies greatly.

As a case in point, some of the inoperable cancers can inflict more pain and suffering than would ever be meted out as punishment for the most heinous crime. Stroke victims who remain partially paralyzed, with personality changes and loss of speech and other important body functions, may live for years in a manner most of us would like to avoid.

The American Heart Association's estimate of costs related to cardiovascular disease for 1980 is $40.8 billion. (See Table 2.) Keep in mind this expenditure is for heart disease *only*, not other serious illnesses. No wonder we feel it is hard to find the money to raise a family, give to world missions, or take a vacation. We are spending it for unnecessary medical care. "Unnecessary" means we could have prevented it!

Did you know that General Motors spends more for employee health care than it does for purchasing the steel to make automobiles? Dr. Michael Debakey, the famous heart surgeon, recently said that prevention is the "only approach" to controlling heart disease. (3) If you are an American male or female, anywhere between the ages of 12 and 102, the odds are very favorable that *your* heart needs a systematic, regular prevention program to guard against heart disease. Forty percent of all heart attack victims die with the first symptom of the heart attack. If you are already dead when the emergency squad comes to help you, all of the latest techniques and cardiac care units will be of no value. That is the strongest reason your heart needs help *now*.

## Heart Risk Factors

To inform you better about your own upkeep, let's take a look at the top ten risk factors of cardiovascular disease, as outlined by the American Heart Association. Some of these risk factors cannot be changed: Heredity, sex, race, age. Some risk factors can be changed by medical supervision: Serum cholesterol, high blood pressure, diabetes, cigarette smoking, diet, stress, and exercise.

1. FAMILY HISTORY. You have a greater chance of heart problems if a blood relative has or had heart disease.

Table 2. Estimated Economic Costs in Billions of Dollars of Cardiovascular Diseases by Type of Expenditure. United States: 1980

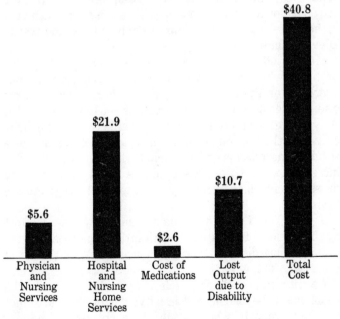

© American Heart Association. Reprinted with permission.

Did your mother or father or a brother or sister die of a heart problem? If the answer is yes, there are steps in other areas you can take to lower your risk situation.

2. EMOTIONAL STRESS AND BEHAVIOR PATTERNS. Tension and stress place high on the list of primary risk factors. Relaxation is necessary to allow our blood pressure to lower after a hard day of tension at the office or at home with the kids. Have you not heard of a football fan becoming so excited watching his son on a Saturday afternoon that he has a heart attack and dies?

Dr. Lawrence Lamb informs us that, "Hardly anyone escapes having a headache. It is man's most common pain, and at least 90 percent of the population experiences headaches at one time or another." Ninety percent of headaches come from emotional stress, he says, and there are 50 billion aspirin-containing tablets consumed each year in the United States. (45) Perhaps we should look for a way to alleviate those stress problems.

Many studies have shown that headaches and tension problems which elevate blood pressure, placing tremendous overloads on the circulatory system, are relieved by exercise. (19, 24, 42, 45) Try it the next time you have a headache. As you begin exercising, you will be able to feel your body relax and the tension headache dissipate. Relief comes as a result of vasodilation (enlargement of the blood vessels). The increased size of the vessels allows a lowering of blood pressure as well as increasing the amount of oxygen to the brain.

3. INACTIVITY. The Framingham Study was an effort by the National Institute of Health to determine risk factors causing heart disease. Inactivity placed third on the list of this study. (42, 43)

As with your skeletal muscles, if you don't exercise the heart muscle beyond normal activity, it atrophies and cannot function properly when needed in a stressful situation. Exercise keeps the heart muscle healthy and enables it to work effectively under most circumstances we humans encounter.

4. HIGH BLOOD PRESSURE. High blood pressure indicates that the blood vessels of the circulatory system are over-stressed during normal function. 120/80 has been set as the ideal blood pressure, but most physicians are not upset when a patient has a reading of 140/90. Hypertension usually is diagnosed if the reading reaches 160/95. (To see how blood pressure affects life expectancy, see Table 3.) Each year more and more people are taking medication to lower their blood pressure and reduce the risk of rupturing a brain blood vessel. Research shows that regular exercise helps control high blood pressure. (6, 9, 19, 29, 41)

Table 3. Blood Pressure and Life Expectancy at Various Ages

| Blood Pressure | Remaining Years | Reduction of Life Expectancy (Years Lost) |
|---|---|---|
| (At Age 35) | | |
| 120/80 | 41½ | |
| 130/90 | 37½ | 4 |
| 140/95 | 32½ | 9 |
| 150/100 | 25 | 16½ |
| (At Age 45) | | |
| 120/80 | 32 | |
| 130/90 | 29 | 3 |
| 140/95 | 26 | 6 |
| 150/100 | 20½ | 11½ |
| (At Age 55) | | |
| 120/80 | 23½ | |
| 130/90 | 22½ | 1 |
| 140/95 | 19½ | 4 |
| 150/100 | 17½ | 6 |

Chart prepared by the Metropolitan Life Insurance Company.

5. ABNORMAL RESTING EKG. Physicians use the resting electrocardiogram (EKG) as a guide to check past performance of the heart muscle in areas such as heart attacks, muscle damage caused by heart attacks, and abnormal heart enlargements.

Most athletes who have competed in track or other exercise activities have a larger heart than normal. The athletic heart is not harmful; it is only the normal response to exercise. The heart grows larger in order to carry on the added demands of strenuous exercise. Physicians are becoming more aware that middle-aged people who were in competitive sports in their youth may possess an enlarged athletic heart and have a varying resting EKG.

The normal male pulse rate is 72 beats per minute (female is 80 beats per minute). Using 72 beats per minute will give us a 24-hour total of 103,680 beats. If, by exercising, the resting pulse rate is lowered to 65 beats per minute, the heart only beats 93,600 times in a 24-hour period—saving 10,080 beats per day. In one year, it saves 3,679,200 beats. What is your resting pulse rate? How much less could your heart be working with a lowered resting pulse rate? Use your calculator—you might be very surprised.

6. OBESITY. Obesity definitely puts more stress on the heart. It must work harder to push blood through the blood vessels because of the pressure placed against the outside of the vessel wall by excess fatty tissue. Ask your son or daughter if he or she would like to walk around with a 30-pound weight strapped to his or her back. Needless to say, it would be uncomfortable, as well as make the heart work harder to carry on normal functions. However, many Christians rationalize that they can be 30 to 60 pounds overweight and still work effectively many hours a day serving the Lord. They are constantly tired.

Life insurance charts show that for an individual 10 pounds overweight at the age of 45, there is an eight percent increase in chance of death. For a person 20 pounds overweight, there is an 18 percent increase; 30 pounds, 28 percent, and 50 pounds, 56 percent. (51) These are FACTS!

Bob Glover and Jack Shepherd, in their new book, *The Runner's Handbook*, make the following observation about the average American.

Too many of us are victims of the disease of inactivity. We are lazy and fat. When Yankee Stadium was remodeled in 1974, it contained 9,000 fewer seats than the old "House that Ruth Built." Why? The seats had to be widened from 18 inches to 22 inches to contain the expanding American posterior! (29)

It has been estimated that your body needs 4000 feet of extra blood vessels to supply nourishment to one pound of fat.

God gave us muscle to enable our bodies to work hard in serving Him. He did provide some fat in our bodies to handle emergency situations that we must face from time to time. God also gave us a brain to be used for logical reasoning. Is it logical to you that you can serve God better with a trim and fit temple?

7. CIGARETTE SMOKING. The American Lung Association informs us that smoke from tobacco contains over 500 known poisons. (15) Among them are carbon monoxide, hydrogen cyanide (a respiratory enzyme poison), pyridine, phenols (cancer-causing agents), aldehydes that irritate the lungs, acrolein (World War I gas), and many hydrocarbons. This smoke (and its accompanying poisons) is absorbed by your lips, oral cavity, and esophagus, and is drawn deep into your lungs. Nicotine irritates the stomach and intestines when swallowed and irritates lung tissue when inhaled.

Cigarette smoking *certainly* is a major cause of heart disease. Even the U.S. Surgeon General admits it. Some authorities place it among the top three causes. (19) The American Heart Association tells us that a person who smokes over two packs of cigarettes a day has three times the likelihood of dying of a heart attack than a nonsmoker. What do you think causes the problem with cigarette smoking? The carbon monoxide in the smoke, like that coming out of automobile exhaust, lowers your red blood cells' capability of carrying oxygen. Red blood cells can carry either oxygen or carbon monoxide, and the monoxide gets first preference.

Our logical God-given brain tells us that the heart of a smoker must pump more blood to get the same amount of oxygen to the muscles and brain. Yet I meet many Christians who somehow find it necessary to smoke, even though they know it is of no benefit to their bodies. Some say, "I really enjoy it and it relaxes me." It is interesting to note that these same individuals have fairly normal blood pressure and resting pulse rates early in the morning. However, after smoking their first cigarette of the day, blood pressure and pulse rate both increase. Nicotine in cigarette smoke increases heart rate as much as 25 beats per minute, makes blood more likely to clot, and constricts blood vessels—all making the heart work harder to get the blood through the vessels. If our heart has to work harder for a habit, does it seem logical to waste extra beats that could be put to better use healthwise?

Did you know that nonsmokers are affected by the smoke they breathe from a smoking friend? Here are a few facts from the American Lung Association:

- Cigarette smoke pollutes air in enclosed places and affects the nonsmoker present.
- Inhaling second-hand smoke makes the heart beat faster, the blood pressure go up, and increases the level of carbon monoxide in the blood.
- There is more cadmium in the smoke that drifts off the burning end of the cigarette than in the drag the smoker takes. Exposure to large doses of cadmium has been related to hypertension, chronic bronchitis, and emphysema.

- Smoke from an idling cigarette contains even more tar and nicotine than smoke directly inhaled.
- The amount of carbon monoxide in the blood of nonsmokers doubles in a poorly ventilated room filled with cigarette smoke. Even outside the room, the inhaled carbon monoxide stays in the body for three or four hours.
- The nonsmoker is forced to breathe in smoke from the burning end of the cigarette as well as the smoke exhaled by the smoker.
- Researchers have found that lung illness is twice as common in young children whose parents smoke at home as compared to those with nonsmoking parents.
- An estimated two million Americans are sensitive to tobacco smoke and suffer smoke-caused asthma attacks.
- The U.S. Surgeon General says, "Nonsmokers have as much right to clean air as smokers have to their so-called right to smoke, which I would redefine as a so-called right to pollute. It is high time to ban smoking from all confined public places such as restaurants, theaters, airplanes, trains, and buses. It is time that we interpret the Bill of Rights for the nonsmoker as well as the smoker." (32)

8. CHOLESTEROL. The Framingham study showed that a male whose cholesterol count goes from 194 to over 250 triples the risk of his first heart attack. (42, 43) (Normal blood cholesterol count is 195-210 mg./100 cc. of blood.) A high level of cholesterol contributes to the formation of fatty plaques along the inside wall of the blood vessels. As the fatty particles build up a layer at a time, the inner diameter of the vessel becomes smaller, slowing the rate of blood flow and making the heart work harder to force the blood through the restricted orifice. The Cooper Aerobics Center in Dallas found that after vigorous aerobic exercise, blood fat levels decrease for a period of 24–36 hours. Dr. Cooper also found that aerobic exercise lowers the cholesterol risk by somehow altering the cholesterol form as it appears in the

bloodstream. (20) Perhaps the exercise prevents fatty particles from building up.

9. TRIGLYCERIDES. Normal triglyceride level is 95-110 mg./100 cc. of blood. Research shows high levels of triglycerides increase heart attack risk. (7, 58, 60, 65, 69) These blood fats are more closely related to intake of starches and carbohydrates than to consumption of eggs, dairy products, and animal fats, which are high in cholesterol.

The level of triglycerides is lowered when we reduce the intake of alcohol, starches, and refined sugar. (Sugar is discussed at length in Chapter 10.) When we eat sugar our liver reacts by manufacturing triglycerides and sending them into the bloodstream. The combined effect of high concentrations of triglycerides and cholesterol is a thickening and slowing down of the blood by these fat globules, causing the fat to adhere readily to the arterial wall.

10. DIABETES. Diabetes, or a familial tendency toward diabetes, is associated with an increased risk of heart attack and stroke. A physician can detect diabetes and prescribe drugs, diet regimens, and weight control with exercise programs to keep it in check.

## Fatigue

This is not listed as a risk factor by the American Medical Association but should be considered as a problem we all face. Fatigue is one of the most common complaints physicians hear when patients tell them of their symptoms. There are many different kinds of fatigue, but to most people it means a sense of exhaustion, weakness, or feeling tired. To some it is an inability to get started or a loss of ability to sustain activity. For others, a short period of work quickly induces fatigue.

Another symptom of fatigue is the loss of ability to concentrate. The loss of energy is often accompanied with irritability. The tired businessman may snap at a member of his family in the evening. Even a child, after a day of too much of everything, may suddenly become cross and irritable when evening approaches. Perceptive parents soon learn to recognize that the child's behavior is a symptom of tiredness.

Many people reach a stage of near-exhaustion before they know they are fatigued. Performance tests prove that their skills diminish and they make more and more mistakes doing simple tasks. The individual is often unaware of his or her mistakes as fatigue progresses.

Fatigue may be a sign of a serious medical problem such as heart disease, cancer, or emotional problems. For a heavy laborer or after strenuous physical activity, it is a natural phenomenon. One of the difficulties in assessing fatigue is that it is so common a part of daily life that it is not always easy to decide whether the fatigue is normal or whether it is an indication of a psychological or physical problem. Normal daily fatigue is many times overcome with regular physical exercise.

### Your Risk Factor Assessment

Cardio-Metrics Inc. has done much in the area of stress testing. Their chart (Table 4) is invaluable in predetermining an individual's heart risk factors before starting an exercise program. (13)

## Table 4. How to Find Out Your Heart Risk

| | | |
|---|---|---|
| **HEREDITY** **1** | No heart disease in family (parents, sisters, brothers only) 1 | One relative over 60 with heart attack 2 |
| **BLOOD PRESSURE** **2** | Low blood pressure 1 | Normal blood pressure or don't know 2 |
| **DIABETES** **3** | Low blood sugar 1 | Normal blood sugar or don't know 2 |
| **SMOKING** **4** | Non-user or stopped permanently 1 | Cigars or pipe only 2 |
| **WEIGHT** **5** | More than 5 lbs underweight 1 | Up to 5 lbs overweight 2 |
| **CHOLESTEROL** **6** | Below 180 1 | 181-205 2 |
| **EXERCISE** **7** | Very active physically in job & recreation 1 | Moderately active in job & recreation 2 |
| **EMOTIONAL STRESS** **8** | No real business or personal pressures 1 | Rare business or personal pressure 2 |
| **AGE** **9** | 10-20 1 | 21-30 2 |
| **SEX AND BUILD** **10** | Female, still menstruating 1 | Male, thin build 2 |

Cross out the box that applies on each line. To score yourself, check the appropriate description for each risk factor. Then add up each row of numbers. Ten to 20 points indicates low risk; 21 to 40, moderate risk; 41 to 60, high risk. Be honest with your selections.

| | | | |
|---|---|---|---|
| Two or more relatives over 60 with heart attack 3 | One relative under 60 with heart attack 4 | Two relatives under 60 with heart attack 5 | Three or more relatives under 60 with heart attack 6 |
| High blood pressure only when upset 3 | Mild high B.P. but no medication needed 4 | High B.P. controlled by by medication 5 | High B.P. not completely controlled by medication 6 |
| Known high sugar controlled by diet 3 | High sugar controlled by tablets 4 | Diabetic on insulin − no complications 5 | Diabetic + complications (circulation, kidneys, eyes) 6 |
| Less than 5 cigarettes daily 3 | 6-20 cigarettes daily 4 | 21-39 cigarettes daily 5 | Over 40 cigarettes daily 6 |
| 6-20 lbs overweight 3 | 21-35 lbs overweight 4 | 36-50 lbs overweight 5 | 51-65 lbs overweight 6 |
| 206-230 or don't know 3 | 231-255 4 | 256-280 5 | Over 281 6 |
| Sedentary job, very active in recreation 3 | Sedentary job, moderately active in recreation 4 | Sedentary job, light recreation exercise 5 | Complete lack of exercise 6 |
| Moderate business or personal pressures 3 | Take pills or drink for stress on occasion 4 | Constantly need pills or drink for stress 5 | Intense problems, can't cope, see psychiatrist 6 |
| 31-40 3 | 41-50 4 | 51-60 5 | Over 60 6 |
| Female, after menopause 3 | Male, average build 4 | Male, fairly stocky 5 | Male, very stocky 6 |

You really need to know what type of heart you have beating in your temple.

Chart prepared by Cardio-Metrics, Inc., 295 Madison Ave., New York, New York 10017. Used by permission.

# CHAPTER 4

## Have a Heart!

The human heart, a magnificent, four-chambered, muscular pump, moves over 4000 gallons of blood through the lungs and out into the body's 75,000 miles of blood vessels each day. To accomplish this huge amount of work, the heart beats over 100,000 times every 24 hours and more than 36 million times per year. The thick muscle of the heart wall contracts to force the blood into circulation, and then relaxes to refill the heart chambers with returning blood.

The heart's action is as close to perpetual motion as any other activity in nature; it works all day and every night for 60, 70, 90, and occasionally even for 100-plus years without stopping. The only rest it gets is a brief fraction of a second between beats. The blood must be forced down into the smallest capillaries, where it supplies all body cells with oxygen and nutrients and removes carbon dioxide and other waste products.

The heart truly is an amazing organ. It should not be taken for granted; each of us has only one. And when it stops, we stop. In view of its tremendous task, we should do all we can to keep our heart healthy.

### What Is a Normal Pulse?

Children have much faster pulse rates than adults. At birth the pulse may be around 130 beats per minute. Normal heart rate for adults is 72 beats per minute for males and 6 to 8 beats per minute faster for the adult female.

Dr. Jeremiah Stamler of Northwestern Medical School

found that males with a resting pulse of over 80 beats per minute had several times the likelihood of dropping dead or having a heart attack as those with rates under 70 per minute. (38) Sudden death occurred 23 times as often for men with resting pulse rates over 80 and high cholesterol levels than for men whose resting pulse rates were below 70 per minute and with low cholesterol levels.

The resting pulse changes in relation to body position. For healthy adult males, the average is 66 beats per minute lying down, 75 seated, and 83 while standing. Your resting pulse increases after eating. The digestive process increases the work of the heart, so a true resting rate is not possible until two or three hours after the last meal. Starvation or a strict diet program usually results in a sharp decrease in heart rate.

## Exercise and Pulse Rate

Exercise stimulates nerve receptors in the muscles. These, through reflex mechanisms, send messages to the brain to speed up the heart. Eventually a number of complex reflexes are involved in speeding up the heart in response to exercise.

The resting pulse rate tends to be slower in physically fit individuals. Before Dr. Roger Bannister (the first human to break the four-minute mile) began training seriously for the big event, his resting pulse rate was in the middle 70's. When he was training, before breaking the world's record, his resting pulse rate was in the middle and high 30's. (38) It is not uncommon for well-conditioned athletes to have resting pulse rates in the low 40's.

The individual who is in good physical condition has only a slight increase in pulse rate with moderate exercise, and the pulse returns to normal after strenuous exercise, usually within two hours. The athlete who stops exercising on a regular basis finds that the longer he is away from exercise the higher his resting pulse rate rises.

Dr. Ralph S. Paffenbarger of the School of Public Health, University of California, Berkeley, studied 16,936 Harvard University alumni ages 35 to 74 over a period of six to ten years. Dr. Paffenbarger found that heart attacks declined with increasing activity. "Strenuous sports showed a strong inverse relation to heart attack risk, while casual sports play was unrelated." Examples of strenuous sports were running, swimming, basketball, handball, and racquetball, while casual sports included games such as golf, bowling, baseball, softball, and volleyball. (50)

Dr. Cheraskin tells us that studies done in Ecuador, Pakistan, and the USSR of people who live well past the age of 100 have shown that a high level of physical activity and low-fat diets are significant common denominators. (16)

In general, if the resting pulse is well over 80, or if it is over 100 two minutes after moderate exercise, the individual is not at an optimal level of fitness and health. Cigarettes, coffee, and stress all increase the pulse. An office worker who drinks several cups of coffee, smokes, fails to get regular exercise, and has office tensions has a fast resting pulse rate and a 20 times higher chance of having a heart attack than his nonsmoking, noncoffee-drinking, and exercising counterpart. Do facts impress you? These are facts!

Speaking of facts, what do insurance companies say about daily habits in relation to life expectancy? Life insurance actuarial standards use many years and thousands of people to arrive at the following statistics:

- You can add *four* years to your life if you *exercise regularly*.
- You can add *five* years to your life if you *don't smoke*.
- You can add *five* years to your life if you practice *weight control* and don't allow yourself to become obese.

- You can add *two* years to your life if you will *eliminate alcohol* from your diet.
- You can add *two* years to your life if you have a *yearly check-up* by your physician. (20)

These measures can add *18 years of life* to your temple, which gives God 18 more years to use your talents. Eighteen years is a chance to relive the length of your childhood all over again, at a later stage in your life.

Insurance companies are not in the business of losing money on those they insure. If you smoke, drink, and are obese, your life-style falls into a certain risk category. The insurance companies know that these risk factors add or take away from human life.

You can lengthen your life by improving your risk potential. I'm sure God wants to use us as long as we are healthy and effective for Him. Philippians 4:8 says:

Finally, brethren, whatever is true, whatever is honorable, whatever is right, whatever is pure, whatever is lovely, whatever is of good repute, if there is any excellence and if anything worthy of praise, let your mind dwell on these things.

Somehow, I cannot help but believe that taking care of ourselves falls within the categories of this passage.

# CHAPTER 5

## Straight Talk About Obesity

Knowledge is the tool we use to choose between right and wrong. The Bible tells us many times to become knowledgeable. In that light, let's find out what God has to say about the abuse of food. Nutrition and diets will be discussed later, but I want to take some time now to mention a few things about overeating.

We talked in Chapter 2 about a general biblical view of ourselves and our bodies. Paul wrote, "Therefore, laying aside falsehood, *speak truth*, each one of you, with his neighbor, for we are members of one another" (Eph. 4:25, italics mine). To begin this chapter, permit me to tell you the truth about overeating. Sometimes fat Christians tell themselves they have some kind of glandular problem or that their thyroid does not work well, even if it's not the truth. Therefore, God won't mind if they are fat.

The truth is almost all overweight people are *foodaholics*. The temptation to overeat now controls them. If you are in this category, I beg you to be honest with yourself. If this is your problem, if you are a foodaholic, I am asking you as plainly as I know how to confess your sin and turn away from it. Listen to Proverbs 23:20,21:

Do not be with heavy drinkers of wine,
Or with gluttonous eaters of meat.
For the heavy drinker and the glutton will come to poverty,
And drowsiness will clothe a man with rags.

God puts the alcoholic and the foodaholic in the same category! Think back for a moment to last Thanksgiving when you spent the day with your family. Or perhaps you were invited by some friends to share their Thanksgiving turkey. Most of us eat way too much on that special day—not one, but usually two plates full of turkey with all of the trimmings. And don't forget the many different desserts that land on your plate.

What do you want to do after gorging yourself? Most of us get very sleepy. So we take a nap to rest up before driving home. We almost always become drowsy after too much food.

This is exactly what Proverbs tells us: Those who are alcoholics or foodaholics become drowsy and, ultimately, lazy. This is why fat people need to deal with their appetites. Not only does obesity cost you your physical health; it affects your spiritual health as well!

Let's ask ourselves some questions concerning being overweight and overfat, and what goes on to turn a healthy body into an unhealthy one. (How does your current weight compare to the "ideal"? See Table 5.)

### Is an Overweight Person an Unhealthy Person?

If God thought fat was a necessary and good thing, would he not have given us *all* excess fat, for energy perhaps? God seemingly created some naturally thin and some potentially fat people. At least, that's how we may view it. But the fact is, almost *every* human being (99.9 percent of us) has the potential to become overweight. Fat, like water, is a good thing, but only in moderation.

The Committee on Exercise and Physical Fitness of the American Medical Association revealed,

One physician who has studied the problems of obesity in great detail says that a woman would need to eat an average of only 96

## Table 5. Ideal Weight Formulas

Ideal body weight can be calculated easily with these formulas.

### WOMEN

1. Multiply your height in inches = _62_ times 3.5 = _217_ and subtract 108= _109_ (**Total or Ideal Weight**)

2. Measure your wrist (at base of hand) in inches = _____ .
   If your wrist is exactly 6 inches, your ideal weight is the same as **Total** above.
   If your wrist is under 6 inches, subtract 10 percent of
   **Total** = _____ from **Total** = _____ . This is your **Ideal Weight**.
   If your wrist is over 6 inches, add 10 percent of
   **Total** = _____ to **Total** = _____ . This is your **Ideal Weight**.

### MEN

1. Multiply your height in inches = _____ times 4 = _____ and subtract 128= _____ (**Total or Ideal Weight**)

2. Measure your wrist (at base of hand) in inches = _____ .
   If your wrist is 6 to 7 inches, your ideal weight is the same as **Total** above.
   If your wrist is under 6 inches, subtract 10 percent of
   **Total** = _____ from **Total** = _____ . This is your **Ideal Weight**.
   If your wrist is over 7 inches, add 10 percent of
   **Total** = _____ to **Total** = _____ . This is your **Ideal Weight**.

### EXAMPLE

1. Author's height in inches = _68_ times 4 = _272_ and subtract _128_ = _144_ (**Total or Ideal Weight**)

2. Author's wrist is over 7 inches. Add 10 percent of
   **Total** = 14 to **Total** = 158. This is author's **Ideal Weight**.

NOTE: As with any weight chart or formula, your ideal weight as calculated above is intended to be only an indicator. The body structure of certain individuals may make the above formulas inaccurate. Your ideal weight should approximate your weight at age 19–21 (assuming you were active during those years).

calories a day more than she expends to gain 50 pounds from the time of her marriage to the arrival of her third child five years later. Had she added only 25 minutes of brisk walking to her daily activities, this weight gain would have been prevented. (4)

So "walk more and eat less" is a rewarding regimen.

## Are We Getting Bigger?

Are we Americans getting bigger? To answer that question, first let us consider the two types of obesity.

1) *Early-onset obesity* begins in childhood, when the *total number* of fat cells is increased. It is estimated that a normal, healthy, lean child has 25 billion fat cells. If a 12-year-old is overweight by 30 to 40 pounds, it is possible that child could develop three to four times the number of fat cells of a healthy child. Needless to say, early-onset obesity is difficult to treat medically in later years because of the extra fat cells present.

It is a shame for parents to allow their children to become fat at a young age. They will most likely have to remain on a constant diet and exercise program throughout their lives to maintain a trim appearance as an adult. I sincerely believe you should safeguard your child's intake of food and insist he exercise at a young age, rather than by default set for him a future trend of getting fatter by the year.

2) The most common type of obesity is *adult-onset obesity*. This obesity pattern is an increase in the *size* of existing fat cells. People with adult-onset obesity gain weight because their caloric intake exceeds their body's ability to burn up the calories. This, as you recall, was my own experience. People lose weight when that process is put into reverse cycle: The body uses up more calories than are put in the mouth.

Although figures on the percentage of the general population that is overweight are relatively sparse, there is good data available on the insured population. (33) Using that weight group which has the lowest death rate as the ideal, half of American men between ages 30 and 39 are at least 10 percent overweight, and a fourth are 20 percent overweight. The percentage of men who are overweight increases with age to approximately 60 years of age.

There are fewer women than men, percentage-wise, who are overweight in their younger years, perhaps because they are more conscious of their appearance. In the middle 40's and beyond, however, the number of overweight women increases until a very high percentage of women past 50 years of age are obese.

As a group, individuals who are obese are *less successful in life*. Many complex factors must be considered to explain this observation. Some individuals who are not successful become fat. They eat out of frustration through years of failed attempts to climb the ladder of success. As a group, individuals who are leaner are more active individuals to begin with. It is possible that the action-oriented individual will be lean and also successful, as opposed to his less action-oriented colleague.

James Trager points out in his recent publication, *The Belly Book*, that a New York personnel agency in 1969 studied 50,000 executive jobs. Of the executives earning $25,000 to $50,000, only 10 percent were more than 10 pounds overweight. Of those individuals in the $10,000 to $20,000 bracket, 35 percent were more than 10 pounds overweight. A representative from the New York personnel agency that conducted the survey was quoted as saying, "The difference between the trim, top-dollar man and his overstuffed, lower-paid colleague may be measured at perhaps $1000 a pound." (63)

The increased obesity in the American population is literally coming out in the end. The American Seating Company has discovered that American seats have expanded nearly two inches in the past 30 years. Information from manufacturers of women's clothing and military organizations indicates that individuals of both sexes, in all ages, show an increase in girth of arms, chest, and body measurements. A higher percentage of women have larger brassiere cups than formerly.

If the American population is actually getting bigger in body size, perhaps we need to learn *why* we are bigger than our forefathers. It is true that the *longer* the *belt*, the *shorter* the *life*.

## Do Fat People Eat Less Than Skinny People?

Most fat people eat less than skinny people *after* they are *already fat!* Through the weight-gaining period most heavy people do eat more than their slender friends. After people become fat and are unhappy with their appearance, they force themselves to eat less food. But this only *maintains* their weight.

By observing men in a prison situation, it has been shown that most heavy people eat less than their skinny friends. (9) Even men who are confined to four prison walls are self-conscious about their weight and eat so as not to gain weight.

Of course, we all know an obese person who keeps gaining weight every year, even though he tells you he is constantly on a diet. This individual usually overeats at each meal and enjoys two or three snacks per day. But we must keep in mind that most, if not all, fat people are unhappy with their excess weight and are affected both mentally and spiritually. This is why people attempt so many diets.

## Is There a Crash Diet That Works?

Some diets do result in weight loss—for a short period of time. Over a long period of time, however, most people go back to their original weight or even get heavier. So the true answer is *no. There is no crash diet that works.* If there was an effective crash diet, there would be no need to print the approximately 20,000 different weight loss programs that are on the market.

An individual who weighs 250 pounds and goes on a diet six times a year probably will not weigh any less at the end of the year than he did at the beginning. He has lost 989 pounds in the last 10 years and now weighs 280 pounds rather than the 250 pounds of 10 years ago. The problem is not losing weight. The problem is gaining weight.

Most diets are composed of two-food regimens. Examples are the grapefruit-egg diet, bananas and milk diet, low carbohydrate-high protein diet. Lopsided diets either aggravate preexisting metabolic imbalances, making them more difficult to correct, or trigger an imbalance where one did not previously exist.

There is a "good news-bad news" aspect of such diets. The good news is that the monotony is apt to bore us into quitting the plan. The bad news is that we may shed weight (how many grapefruits can you eat and stay healthy?) and thereby be encouraged to continue to ruin our health. We have all seen the individual who sticks to a two-food diet and the gray, sick look he takes on as a result.

Physicians are often accused of contributing to obesity by encouraging patients to go on special diets, with or without drugs. The patients lose a few pounds, but after the doctor tells them what a nice job they have done, three months later they weigh *more* than when they first visited the doctor. Fat people who crash diet are in reality getting fatter.

It is not the doctor who is to blame; rather obesity is not clearly addressed. If patients would return to their physicians for several months after attaining their desired weight, perhaps more success could be achieved. Instead, after an initial loss the patient soon eats himself to a heavier weight. One year later he returns to the doctor, 15 pounds heavier than when he first went on a diet.

Losing excess poundage is actually the easiest part of a weight reduction program. *Keeping it off* is the hardest battle. There are three main ingredients to successful dieting: calorie restriction (Chapter 10), exercise (Chapter 6), and behavior modification (Chapter 13). If one of these is lacking, a weight loss program simply won't work.

## What Does *Metabolism* Mean?

Metabolism is your body's ability to use the food you eat and break it down into energy for your body. Metabolism utilizes protein, carbohydrate, and fat from our food to enable us to function.

Most people want to lose fat, not muscle tissue, when they go on a diet. Your muscles provide your basic strength and are the energy cells of your body. During physical exercise, energy is released inside the muscle cell. There is no evidence that a heavy muscular body is unhealthy. The health problems from body weight are associated with an excess accumulation of *fat*. If a person needs to lose weight, it is important that he do so without losing muscle mass. Severe dieting imposes a risk of loss of muscle mass in addition to loss of fat.

There is no place for the *total fast diet* (only water and vitamin supplements for days). (28) The appearance of men released after they have been prisoners of war is obviously unhealthy. When the body needs energy to survive, it metabolizes muscle if the fat available is insufficient.

It was shown by F. G. Benedict in 1915, and again very recently by a group of Georgetown University physicians, that in starvation diets 50 percent of the weight loss is muscle mass. (37) Can you afford to lose 50 percent of your "burning machine" of calorie intake? Loss of lean body mass is not the only problem with fasting. Psychological problems as well as disruption of normal organ function have been documented during prolonged days of fasting. (28)

My sincere desire is that no one use a starvation diet to attempt weight loss. I also do not recommend that an orthodontist wire your mouth shut to prevent you from eating. God's discipline is vastly superior! A dieting temple cannot be healthy when 50 percent of the loss is God-given muscle mass.

Many fad diets have an effect similar to starvation. To avoid muscle loss while on a diet, it is best to consume at least 1000 calories a day, and to include from 40 to 70 grams of protein. The best way to insure further that you don't lose muscle mass is to use a suitable exercise program while dieting.

Dr. Zuti and Dr. Golding reported a very interesting study in the January 1976 issue of *Physician and Sports Medicine*. They studied three groups of women, 20 to 40 pounds overweight. The study lasted for 16 weeks. The Zuti-Golding study is a classic. I urge you to look at the results carefully. (69)

GROUP 1. *Diet group*. Reduced daily caloric intake 500 calories below the amount needed to maintain present body weight (normal metabolic rate). Example: If 2000 calories kept one of the ladies at her present weight, then her caloric intake was cut to 1500 calories.

GROUP 2. *Exercise group*. Increased their physical activity to expend 500 calories a day while staying on a diet that maintained their present body weight (normal metabolic rate).

GROUP 3. *Combined group*. Increased their physical activity to expend 250 calories per day and decreased their food intake by 250 calories per day (normal metabolic rate).

Each group altered the diet needed to maintain weight by a total of 500 calories per day.

GROUP 1. Lost an average of 11.7 pounds of weight. (They lost 9.3 pounds of fat *plus* 2.4 pounds of *muscle*).

GROUP 2. Lost an average of 10.6 pounds of weight. They *lost* 12.6 pounds of fat but *gained* 2.0 pounds of *muscle*).

GROUP 3. Lost an average of 12 pounds of weight. (They *lost* 13.0 pounds of fat *plus gained* 1.0 pounds of *muscle*).

Both the exercise (Group 2) and the combination diet-exercise (Group 3) groups increased muscle and lost more body fat than Group 1, which dieted only and lost muscle as well as fat. The study clearly demonstrates that exercise is effective in preventing the loss of body protein which is evident in dieting without exercise.

An interesting aspect of the study is that the dieting group lost a total of 33,990 calories, the exercise group lost 43,980 calories, and the combination group lost 44,900 calories total even though all of the groups reduced their daily caloric intake by only 500 calories. Using a scale of 3,500 calories for a pound of body fat and 600 calories for a pound of gained or lost lean body mass, you will observe there is a *greater* loss of calories in those who *combine* diet with exercise. The calories lost must be the difference between the calories used by the body and the calories consumed since energy can neither be created nor destroyed.

When it is stated that a certain exercise uses up 10 calories per minute, say in jogging, the figure applies only to the time during which the individual is exercising. The Zuti-Golding study clearly shows that the total calories used for exercising was *greater* than the value assigned for the activity. The increase in metabolism after physical exercise *may actually persist for hours*, burning up more calories after the exercise is completed.

The lesson in all of these facts is that you will get better results and have a better, healthier, and firmer body if you *combine* your diet program with a sensible exercise program.

Dieting without changing an individual's metabolism will not work. You can diet your way into disaster, or you can diet your way into optimal physical and mental health. You make the choice. It's your temple that God is lending you to use.

All of the energy used to run your body ultimately comes from the sun. The energy is locked in the food you eat and the process of metabolism releases the energy so you can use it to grow body cells, do physical activities for work or play, and in general run your body. Energy can neither be created nor destroyed, but it can be transformed. Your energy system literally transforms the energy in your food to give you energy for body functions. It is little wonder, then, that if there is a defect in the ability to release energy from food, you feel tired.

When a healthy person eats 1000 calories, all of the calories are burned up. When a fat person eats 1000 calories, approximately 900 of them are used up. The remaining 100 are converted to fat. The metabolism of an obese person converts food into fat storage more easily than in the healthy person. Covert Bailey, in his book, *Fit or Fat*, feels the reason a fat person converts more ingested food into fat storage is because he or she has different enzymes in his or her bloodstream. (9)

## How Do Muscles Work?

To understand exercise it's important that we understand muscles, for it is through muscle function that we actually accomplish exercise. The body has three types of muscles: (1) *voluntary* or *skeletal* muscles, such as the biceps, found in the upper arm, (2) *involuntary* muscles, such as those found in the digestive tract, and (3) the *heart* muscle. In exercise we concentrate on the use of voluntary muscles.

Approximately 45 percent of a healthy person's body weight is muscle. Each muscle is made up of millions of individual muscle fibers. Muscle fibers contain a small amount of fat, but they are mainly composed of protein. Fat between the muscle protein fibers does not contribute in muscle contraction. Fat actually causes friction in the muscle and makes for more difficult contraction.

To maintain normal function and make contractions possible, the muscle fibers must have food, in the form of carbohydrates and fats, as well as oxygen. *Protein is not used for muscle contraction.* Eating high protein foods, such as meat, to provide fuel or energy to cause muscles to work is a fallacious concept.

Protein eaten in the diet is processed by the liver and converted to carbohydrate or fat which then becomes the necessary fuel for muscle function, or it is stored as body fat.

Protein is necessary and important for growth, including formation of muscles; it is not essential as fuel for muscular contraction.

Fat is processed by the muscle fibers to form carbon dioxide and water. *Fat, however, is a very small part of the fuel for muscular contraction.*

### How Is Energy Stored in Muscles?

Carbohydrates are stored in the muscle fibers in the form of glycogen. Glycogen is a long series of glucose molecules. Glucose is the simple sugar used by the muscle for fuel. Glucose is a carbohydrate and makes up the vast majority of fuel for muscle contraction.

The use of glucose and fat to produce energy within the muscle fiber releases a great amount of heat. Almost 40 percent of the energy of muscular activity is dissipated as heat. The heat warms the skin; thus muscular activity is a major source of body heat. Thus if we move quickly, causing increased muscular heat, our body temperature increases.

## How Do Muscles Grow?

Growth of muscles and contraction of muscles are entirely two different things. Muscle contraction uses carbohydrates (glucose) for fuel. For a muscle to grow it must have amino acids provided from proteins. Muscle growth occurs primarily during an individual's developmental years, usually up to 18 years of age; muscle contraction continues throughout our lives.

There are chemical factors which influence the cellular machinery in producing muscle growth. Some of these are thyroxin, the growth hormone; thyroglobulin, the thyroid hormone; and the male hormone, testosterone. It is no accident that men tend to develop a larger, more defined muscle mass than women. This effect is a direct result of the action of testosterone upon the growth mechanism of the man's muscles. Women can gain muscular strength by exercising, but they usually do not develop large masses of muscle because they lack the male hormone. So, ladies, don't tell us you can't exercise because it will give you big leg muscles!

Just as work or exercise leads to the development of muscles, lack of physical activity leads to a decrease in muscle size and loss of muscle mass. One of the best examples of this is the results of prolonged bed rest. When muscles are not used, they decrease in size and muscle protein is actually destroyed. The excess nitrogen shows up in the patient's urine. As the muscle tissue degenerates the interior of the muscle becomes infiltrated with fat. By replacing the muscular structure with fat the muscles become increasingly ineffective.

Individuals who have been relatively inactive will develop increased muscle mass once they start engaging in regular physical activity.

## Can Body Chemistry Be Altered to Convert Less Calories?

Most of us operate on the assumption that there are people

who get fat easily and people who stay underweight regardless of what they eat. This assumption definitely is not true. Don't we all have a friend who was skinny as a child and who now can't seem to control his weight? Is there a way to alter our body chemistry? The answer is yes! The only proven way to alter our body chemistry is through exercise and proper diet which allows for *slow weight loss*.

Physicians tell us that we should actually weigh less at age 30 than we weighed at age 18. How many people do you know who weigh less now than when they were in high school? Most American adults weigh 20 to 30 pounds more at age 30 than they weighed on graduation day.

### Is It Possible to be Overfat but Not Overweight?

A person who is not fat in appearance, but who has an inefficient muscle machine, may have fatty tissues. His body chemistry burns up the calories he eats, but his muscles are infiltrated with fatty deposits.

### How Can We Be Fit and Not Fat?

The solution to the problem of fat is simple, but it takes a change in attitude. We must develop an attitude of changing our muscles into efficient eight-cylinder machines instead of sloppy, four-cylinder putt-putts. The answer is, *We must exercise our muscles*.

In *Fit or Fat*, Covert Bailey says that if you are only five pounds overweight it is probable that you are 13 pounds *overfat*. (9)

In order to learn how we can change our muscle content, we need to understand the term *lean body mass* (LBM). (2, 30) LBM is the weight of muscle, bones, and organs, minus the weight of fat. LBM can be determined by weighing a person on a scale and then dipping that person in a water tank to find out how much that person weighs underwater. Since fat floats, it does not weigh underwater. The more fat you have on your body the better you will be able to float in a swimming pool.

The amount of LBM you have determines how much you should eat. LBM, which is mainly muscle, burns up the majority of calories we eat. Fat is not part of the LBM. *Fat on our body does not burn up calories* but is a storehouse for the excess calories our muscles don't burn up.

Bailey says, after testing hundreds of people, that the average American male is made up of 23 percent body fat and the average American female is 32 percent body fat. (9) Dr. Ken Cooper's clinic reports the average male at 26 percent body fat and female at 34 percent. He also feels that the normal, healthy male should be 15–17 percent body fat and the female should be 22–24 percent body fat. (20)

Average and normal should not be confused. The athlete with six percent body fat is included with the 300-pound "hippo" who has 55 percent body fat to give us an average. I found it interesting that the average female student tested by Ohio State University's Exercise Physiology Department was 25-28 percent body fat, while the average male tested was 12-14 percent body fat. (26) It appears that our female students entering college are fatter by 20 years than their mothers. Most mothers do not approach 30 percent body fat until they reach 40-49 years of age. Perhaps we should think about where our percent of body fat *should be* rather than simply being relieved if we are at the low end of the average American fat scale.

### Turning Fat into Muscle

The degree of athletically trained muscle present in our bodies appears to determine the amount of food we can eat. As muscle turns to fat, not only does the actual size of muscles decrease, thereby decreasing the need for calories, but also the chemistry of the remaining muscle changes in such a way as to use less calories.

Dieting may decrease your excess fat, but it cannot increase the amount of muscle or reverse the badly altered chemistry of the non-exercised muscle. By failing to exercise properly we cheat our hearts of improvement in heart-lung endurance and in oxygen consumption capacity (fitness). We cheat ourselves of the opportunity to feel better, look better, cope with stress better, overcome mental and physical fatigue more quickly, and perform better in all areas of life.

Having lived in Ohio my entire life, I am a fan of the Ohio State Buckeyes football team. For sports fans who follow the Buckeyes, it is obvious that "that state up North" (Michigan) is our big rival. I was recently asked if I knew the definition of the action taking place during an Ohio State-Michigan football game. The answer was: 22 men on the field desperately in need of rest, and 85,000 people watching the game in desperate need of exercise.

# CHAPTER 6

## Exercise: God's Fat-Abatement Plan

To be beneficial, any physical activity, according to the President's Council on Physical Fitness and Sports, should be "vigorous enough to tax the power of the muscles and should be done long enough and strenuously enough to produce a sense of healthful fatigue." (55)

The type of exercise that builds this fitness is *aerobic*, so-called because it increases oxygen-consumption capacity. Aerobic means "oxygen-in-air." Aerobic exercise demands a steady output from your muscles over a long period of time. Jogging, cycling, racquetball, and tennis are all good examples. One can participate in aerobic exercise in a continuous, steady-state manner for 15, 20, 30, or 60 minutes without stopping. Even walking is an aerobic exercise. It produces a good training effect if done frequently enough, briskly enough, and for a long enough period of time.

One of the best cures for obesity is aerobic exercise. (7, 19, 54) It has been shown in many exercise physiology laboratories that steady, continuous exercise repeated each day quickly reverses the syndrome of muscle turning to fat. (54)

### Long Slow Distance

Joe Henderson, consulting editor of *Runner's World Magazine*, popularized the term *long slow distance* (LSD). (39, 57) Long slow distance jogging is the best aerobic exercise. We should jog at a pace which is 80 percent of our maximum heart rate or that pace at which you can carry on a conversation as you jog. (How to determine your maximum heart rate and your 80 percent rate is discussed in Chapter 9.)

Covert Bailey feels you can get as much benefit from 15 minutes of jogging as from two hours of tennis. (9) (We are speaking here of cardiopulmonary "heart-lung" exercise). Dr. Ken Cooper feels you must play two and one-half hours of tennis to get the same aerobic benefit as 18 minutes of jogging. (19) (See Table 6.) You can make your muscles lean by playing tennis, but you will have to play hard for two and one-half hours a day for five days each week. Most people do not have enough time or money to play tennis for 12½ hours per week. Can you think of a friend who plays tennis two times a week but seems to stay 20 pounds overweight?

Table 6. The Aerobic Value of Various Sports

| 18 minutes of jogging is equal to:* | |
| --- | --- |
| 30 minutes of | swimming |
| 38 minutes of | rope skipping |
| 40 minutes of | cycling |
| 45 minutes of | continuous stair climbing |
| 50 minutes of | stationary running |
| 60 minutes of | racquetball |
| 1 hour 20 minutes of | stationary cycling |
| 1 hour 45 minutes of | snow skiing |
| 1 hour 45 minutes of | football |
| 2 hours 15 minutes of | ice or roller skating |
| 2 hours 30 minutes of | volleyball |
| 2 hours 30 minutes of | tennis |
| 18 hours of | golf |

*Dr. Ken Cooper gives this information in his book, *The Aerobic Way*, but uses aerobic points rather than time periods. (One aerobic point is equal to 7 milliliters of oxygen per kilogram body weight/minute. Aerobic points are not strictly rate measurements but are dependent upon the intensity and duration of the activity.)

An *anerobic* exercise is intense but short, requiring little oxygen. When a football lineman charges across the scrimmage line to hit his opponent, he is basically doing anerobic exercise. The short, extreme, sudden burst of energy does not require a lot of oxygen; the muscle mass gets its energy from glucose in the muscle.

An aerobic exercise is less intense but longer lasting, requiring significant oxygen.

Aerobic running will get you into shape for an anerobic sport (tennis, handball), but an anerobic exercise will not get you into shape for an aerobic exercise (jogging or running for long periods of time).

If we run a quarter of a mile as fast as we can, our bodies burn up all of the glucose in the bloodstream. If we continue to run, the body must produce more glucose for the muscle cells to burn. How does the body make new glucose under stress? It breaks down protein and turns it into energy, and the most available protein is muscle tissue. However, if we run slower, at a jogging pace, the body breaks down subcutaneous and intramuscular fat into glucose, instead of muscle. So it appears to be common sense that an aerobic exercise is the best exercise for people who are not engaged in competitive athletics.

### Jogging

Many times I am asked, "Why do you jog?" My reply usually includes these reasons:

1. It is something we can do for ourselves.
2. It costs little money.
3. It can be done when I plan for it.
4. It makes me feel good for many hours after doing it.
5. I know my temple is healthier for having done it.

About the only risk of jogging as a regular exercise is that you miss it very much when you don't do it. Those people who jog regularly are very upset if they miss three days in a row.

Did you know there are an estimated 20-25 million *regular joggers* in America today? Do you notice how many more joggers you see today in the morning hours, at lunchtime, and in the evening than you saw five years ago? You can be added to the ranks. Both jogging and walking briskly are natural and easy. Both are economical. You don't have to join a country club, make a reservation at the park, or pay a fee to anyone.

Long slow distance is the exercise I recommend. If you have not exercised for a period of time and have *permission from your physician*, it is time to start a jogging program. I would suggest that an exercise of 12-15 minutes per day be started as soon as you finish this book and really have a true handle on aerobic exercise. Of course someone who is really overfat or quite out-of-shape may reach 80 percent maximum heart rate by a fast walk rather than by jogging.

Most women do not want to jog around a track with people watching them. Many women who are overweight do not want to have other people, especially their husbands, watching them. So ladies, I have a suggestion for you. Why don't you set a goal of jogging indoors for six minutes per day?

If possible run a circular course (which is easier on your knees and ankles) inside your house or basement. Perhaps you can run from the kitchen to the family room to the living room, through the foyer into the dining room, and back to the kitchen. That was my wife's path in our house during the winter months before we joined a health club. It is recommended that you jog six days per week and rest one day, preferably Sunday.

If you ladies increase each week's running *by only one minute per day*, you will be able to run one hour per day in only a year. Most people don't have an hour a day to exercise, but we surely can find 20-30 minutes per day for our temple upkeep. Maybe due to your physical condition you can't start out jogging 20 minutes per day, but that is a reasonable goal that *almost everyone* can attain within six months' time.

Unfortunately, most of us men have tremendous ego problems associated with exercising. We get on the track and our minds think back to when we were trained athletes. We run fast and hard for eight minutes and then go sit down and gasp for air, hoping we impressed everyone on the track with how hard we worked. Unfortunately, we accomplished very little aerobically or in terms of burning up fat. At the end of eight minutes we have used up blood glucose and probably have lost muscle because we needed more glucose than was present in our bloodstream.

Since our brain is smarter than our ego, it signals the body to convert muscle protein to needed blood glucose. So we leave the track barely sweating, with less muscle, same amount of fat as before our ego trip, and think we have exercised. In fact we have done more anerobic than aerobic exercise, and since our bodies are not well-conditioned to stress, we have really done more harm than good. Getting a stress electrocardiogram before you begin stressful exercise is definitely recommended.

## Benefits of Aerobic Exercise

1. Aerobic exercise increases the amount of blood in your system and increases the amount of oxygen-carrying hemoglobin in the blood. The blood is able to carry more oxygen to each cell and take away more carbon dioxide. Your muscle cells improve their ability to process the oxygen and eliminate wastes more efficiently. Consequently, your heart doesn't have to pump as much blood to each cell as it did before.

2. Aerobic exercise increases the working space and efficiency of your lungs and strengthens the muscles that make your lungs expand and contract.

3. Aerobic exercise makes your blood vessels more flexible, so that they tend not to accumulate arteriosclerotic deposits as readily; consequently, less resistance in the blood vessels and less work for your heart.

4. Aerobic exercise increases the number of tiny blood vessels that form a network throughout the cells of your body.

Exercise is becoming more accepted by physicians as part of the rehabilitation program for anyone who has had a heart attack or blood vessel problem. BUT—*if you have a history of heart disease, DON'T read this book and begin exercising without getting medical clearance.* This book does not explain the many extenuating circumstances of heart disease.

Your physician may want to place you on a program of walking before you engage in an aerobic jogging exercise program. If the doctor feels your heart will not allow you to walk, then I suggest you get a second opinion—for your health's sake. I feel that future studies will show that proper diet and proper exercise are the answers to heart attack recovery. The Framingham study found sedentary people have more than double the cardiac mortality rate of people in the active category. (42, 43)

## Heart and Circulation

The beneficial effects of exercise on the heart and circulation are primarily achieved by stimulating the heart to pump more blood than it does during resting (normal function or sleeping). The heart is no different than any other muscle in the body. If it is not used to its full range of function, it will lose its capacity. It's like the old story: If you don't use it, you will lose it.

Exercise requires more oxygen to be delivered to the working muscles. Unless the exercise requires a great amount of oxygen, it has little or no effect in maintaining the functional capacity of the heart and circulation. Any exercise which involves only a small group of muscles, whether it be isometric (muscle tensing; push-resist stress) or isotonic (movement with muscles shortening and lengthening; lifting weights), has little effect upon the heart and circulation. The larger the number of muscle groups exercised, the more oxygen the heart and circulation must deliver. If you open and close your hand rapidly, the muscles of the hand become fatigued. But due to the small number of muscles involved, the exercise has basically no effect on the heart or circulation.

Under resting conditions in an adult man, the body requires as little as a half pint of oxygen each minute for the cells of the entire body. During exercise, such as jogging, the body requires as much as four quarts of oxygen a minute. To deliver this amount of oxygen to the muscles and cells, the heart pumps up to 30 quarts of blood a minute. At rest the heart usually pumps only about five quarts of blood per minute.

Regular, vigorous levels of exercise increase the volume capacity of the heart. In sedentary persons the heart tends to be small and its total capacity to hold blood is limited (volume is low). During physical exercise, when the heart is repeatedly called upon to deliver more oxygen to the working muscles, its capacity increases (volume is high). The large pumping chambers of the heart increase in size. Many athletes have hearts twice the size (volume capacity) of sedentary individuals.

As we know, the heart is a muscle. God designed the heart muscle to beat automatically and work without undue fatigue, even though it is not afforded a long-term resting period. But the *heart still is a muscle*, with some characteristics similar to skeletal muscle.

The work of the biceps muscle, as an example, is greater if it must lift 75 pounds through a distance of one foot than if it lifts only five pounds through a distance of one foot. The heart muscle works in a similar manner. The amount of blood that the heart must pump at a given pressure determines how much work the heart muscle must do. Just as increased work of skeletal muscles requires more oxygen to work, increased work of the heart muscle also requires more oxygen. Regular exercise increases the circulation to the heart muscle, thereby enabling the heart to work harder to deliver more oxygen to the working body muscles.

It is not necessary to undergo exhausting physical exercise to develop good circulation. Most studies suggest that regular *moderate* exercise is the best means. Animal studies, as well as studies done on patients with various heart problems that increase the work of the heart, confirm that *increased work of the heart muscle increases its blood supply.* (47)

During reasonable vigorous physical activity, the blood pressure increases. The increased amount of blood being pumped into the arterial system by the heart is chiefly responsible for the rise in pressure. A sedentary person who has a resting blood pressure of 120/80 may have a blood pressure of 200/115 during physical exercise. *With training* the diastolic, or lower reading, usually does not rise very much during exercise. After improving his physical condition this same individual might have a blood pressure of 200/85 during the same level of exertion. The difference between a diastolic pressure of 115 and 85 is that the heart has to do much less work. Even in individuals in good physical condition, the systolic, or upper reading, rises sharply.

With improved fitness a reflex mechanism develops to open or dilate the innumerable small arteries in the working muscles. This way the increased amount of blood that is pumped by the heart into the arterial system runs off rapidly and allows the diastolic reading to fall to levels commonly observed at rest. In healthy individuals the blood pressure quickly returns to normal levels shortly after exercise stops. Many human studies show that regular physical exercise results in lowering of the individual's blood pressure. If your blood pressure is lower, you have less chance of blowing a hole in an artery or heart wall when in a stressful situation.

## Circulatory Efficiency

Something that is often overlooked when considering circulation of blood is *circulatory efficiency*. (36) Regular physical exercise improves circulatory efficiency. Remember that circulation is very much like a complex plumbing system: The arteries represent many pipes that end up in small arteries that are multiple faucets. By constricting arteries in one region in the body and opening arteries to other regions in the body, the proportions of blood that are sent to different parts of the body can be controlled.

For example, if you exercise a person on a treadmill with one arm held stationary, the blood flow to the resting arm markedly decreases, even compared to its level during rest, while the exercise is in progress. The arteries to the stationary arm are constricted and the arteries to the working legs are opened, thereby sending the majority of blood pumped by the heart to the working leg muscles.

Why is the efficiency of circulation important? If a sedentary individual runs to catch a bus, which is an unusual effort for that body, the circulatory system will not be able to shunt the major portion of the increased blood flow to his leg muscles. Instead, a large portion of the blood will continue to flow to non-working muscles in the arms and elsewhere in the body. This is very inefficient. In such an individual blood may have to be pumped twice as fast as in an individual who is in good physical condition. The blood flow to his heart muscle may have to be doubled. If he already has some changes in his coronary arteries to the heart muscle, this may not be possible and running to catch a bus *for him* may cause a heart attack.

By contrast, in the individual accustomed to jogging, with adequate circulatory efficiency, a major portion of the blood pumped by the heart will easily be shunted to his working leg muscles and the work of the heart will be increased only a small amount. Such an individual's heart is in better condition to withstand an increased work load than in the sedentary person. A general rule in physical fitness is to maintain a level of fitness well above the peak loads of physical effort that may be required in ordinary life stress situations.

In developing circulatory efficiency it must be pointed out that this is achieved through *gradual* conditioning of complex reflex mechanisms. The development of the nerve pathways that enable shutting down the arteries in one part of the body and opening those to others requires time and training, just as it requires time to train the nerve mechanisms to play a piano.

### Work and Exercise: Any Difference?

Carrying clothes to the basement to be washed, picking up after the kids all day, washing dishes, or scrubbing the floor will make you very tired, but it is not exercise; just as dad working long hours sitting at his desk using up brain energy is not exercise; both are considered work. With all of the above activities, very little continual effort is expended even though we are exhausted at the end of the day. Exercise is a continual, steady working of the muscles over a period of time. If we carried the clothes from the second floor to the basement and back to the second floor without stopping for 18 minutes, that would be exercise.

# CHAPTER 7

## Getting Started on Weight Control

Before listing guidelines for getting started on weight control, perhaps I should interject my own philosophy about starting an exercise program. The lesson to be learned about exercise is that it must be treated with respect.

Exercise can be compared to a medicine you might take; it can help you or it can harm you. You wouldn't take a whole bottle of aspirin for a headache. The same is true with exercise.

The people who get into trouble with exercise are those who foolishly disregard the proper initiation of exercise. No one can guarantee you that by following any set of rules you won't have a heart attack during or immediately after exercise. But, no one can guarantee that you won't have one in your sleep, either.

### Guidelines for Exercise

If you follow the sensible guidelines set forth here, you will minimize your chances that exercise will be an important factor in causing a heart attack.

#### Have a Check-up

This is probably the most important part of any exercise program. Most physicians are equipped to take a resting EKG. It is important that your physician do a stress EKG if you are over 35 years of age with a family history of heart disease. Based on your past medical history, your present health condition, and your stress EKG, your physician will determine if you should proceed.

If you are obese, there is a very good chance your physician will limit your exercise to walking and restrict your diet until you have lost sufficient weight to allow you to be placed on a jogging program.

But whatever your condition, once you get your physician's approval—*Start immediately!*

## Warm Up Slowly and Thoroughly

No matter who you are, a well-conditioned athlete or sometime jogger, you need a good warm-up period before getting involved in vigorous exercise. Warm-up helps guard against cramps, sprains, strains, and shin splints. Without a warm-up, any resting heart, if instantaneously stressed, will show signs of insufficient blood supply.

Stretching a muscle properly means stretching it slowly. This cannot be done by bobbing or jerking motions, such as bouncing downward to touch your toes. Such action will actually tighten the muscle instead of stretching it.

On the following pages are drawings of stretching exercises that will warm you up effectively for aerobic activities. Instructions are listed with each illustration. Stretching is not a contest and should be fun. Again, DON'T BOUNCE! The proper stress points for each exercise are indicated in most illustrations by black circle(s). NOTE: All of these exercises can be done by men; some of them will be more difficult for women. EVERYONE SHOULD USE CAUTION AND GOOD JUDGMENT.

## Food and Exercise Don't Mix

You should avoid exercising for at least three hours after eating. After a big meal your blood is diverted away from your brain and heart muscle to your stomach to help digest the food.

I find it easier to run early in the morning before breakfast to avoid the digesting problem. However, my son, Rob, feels he can exercise better if he has eaten and allowed his blood glucose level to increase. It is a personal preference, and you should find what works best for you. Many people prefer a glass of fruit juice about fifteen minutes before jogging. The juice, being a carbohydrate, causes an increased blood glucose level.

## When to Exercise

We are all busy and must find time for our new habit. The trick lies in knowing where to find the time. Each of us has a different schedule. It may be easier for you to select a certain time of the day, each day, that will allow you to run.

The easiest time of the day for me to jog, the time least likely to be disrupted by unexpected intrusions, is early in the morning. I get up at 5:00 A.M., floss and brush my teeth, shave, and get my jogging gear on by 5:15 A.M. Then I read the Bible from 5:15 to 5:40 A.M., when my wife and I leave for the Worthington High School track. We arrive at the track usually by 5:50 A.M., do warm-up and stretching exercises, and then run a predetermined length of time. Usually we are back home by 7:00 to 7:15 A.M., leaving enough time for me to shower and eat breakfast before getting to the office by 8:00 A.M.

Some people don't like to get up early, not even for health reasons. If you fall into that category, try to fit your exercise program in at lunchtime. Lunchtime is a good second choice as it gives you added energy for the afternoon work load.

If lunchtime does not permit you to run and take a shower, you may choose to run after work. Running after work has advantages. It is the best time to get rid of the day's tensions. Exercise diminishes your appetite and keeps you from eating too much dinner. There is no reason not to run in the park after dinner at night, as long as the footing is good,

*(Continued on page 96.)*

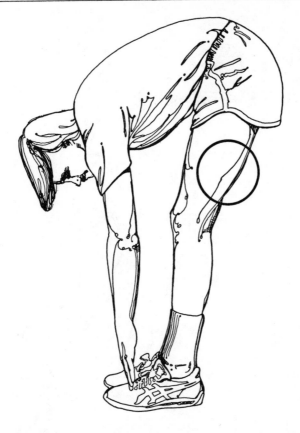

HAMSTRINGS. Start in a standing position. Keep feet as wide as shoulders; bend slowly at the waist. With knees fairly rigid, bend as far as you can and hold for 15–20 seconds. (A slight pulling effect will be felt in the back of the legs.) WITHOUT BOUNCING, reach closer to the ground as the hamstrings loosen. Hold this position for 15–20 seconds. Reach further, as close to the ground as possible and hold for another 15–20 seconds. *CAUTION:* After stretching the hamstrings, DO NOT return to the upright position with knees straight. While bending over, *bend knees slightly* before standing erect. This will put less pressure on back and prevent weakening back muscles.

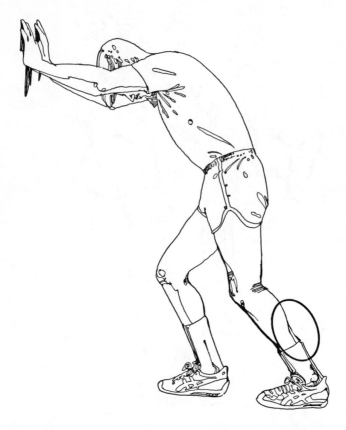

CALF MUSCLE AND ACHILLES TENDON. Stand 3–4 feet from vertical surface with feet together. Place hands on surface about shoulder level. (Rest forearms instead if more comfortable.) Place right foot 12 inches ahead of left foot. Bend right knee and bring it toward surface. Keep left leg straight and heel of left shoe flat on floor. Point toes straight ahead. Place pressure on right leg, keeping left foot flat. The more right knee is bent, the greater will be the tension in calf muscle and Achilles tendon of left leg. Hold for 20–30 seconds. Switch leg positions. Do each leg twice. *This is a very important exercise for joggers.*

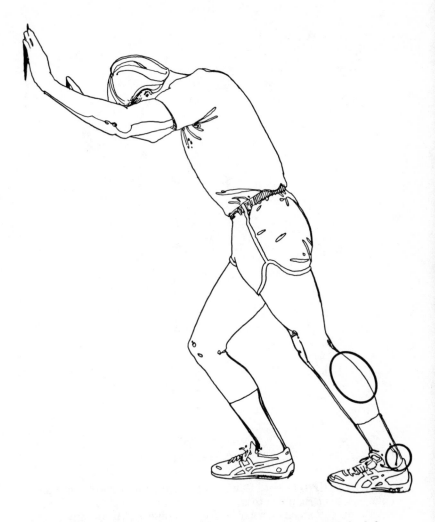

CALF MUSCLE AND ACHILLES TENDON. Next, bend the left
knee to stretch further the Achilles tendon. Lean forward as far as
possible. Hold for 20–30 seconds. Switch leg positions.

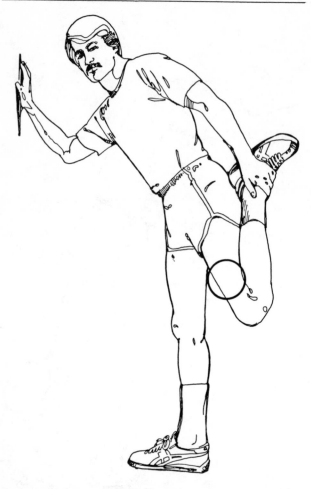

QUADRICEPS (Thighs). Stand 3–4 feet away from a vertical surface. Put weight on right foot to start with and lean with right hand against the surface. Right arm should be fairly straight with body fairly erect. Using the left hand, grab left foot and pull it toward buttocks until stretching is felt in quadriceps. Slowly rotate trunk to give more benefit from exercise. Stretch for 20–30 seconds. Switch legs.

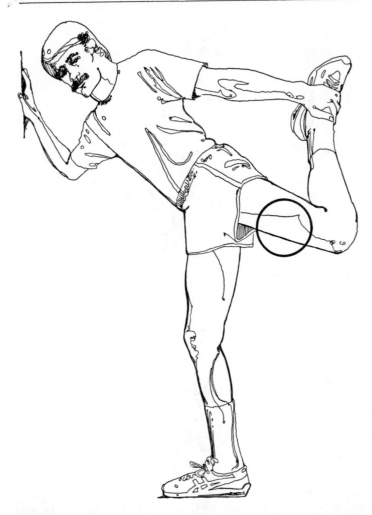

QUADRICEPS. To do next stretch, simply straighten left leg still standing erect and grasping the ankle with left hand. This intensifies stretching in left quadricep. Stretch in this position only 10–15 seconds. Switch legs.

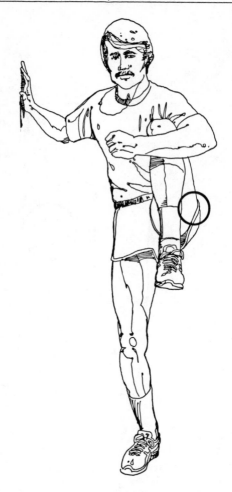

HAMSTRINGS (while standing). Pull knee toward chest, keeping balance by leaning against a vertical surface. This will stretch hamstring and buttock muscles. Keep back straight. Don't jerk, but apply steady pressure to knee. Stretch at least 30 seconds. Switch legs.

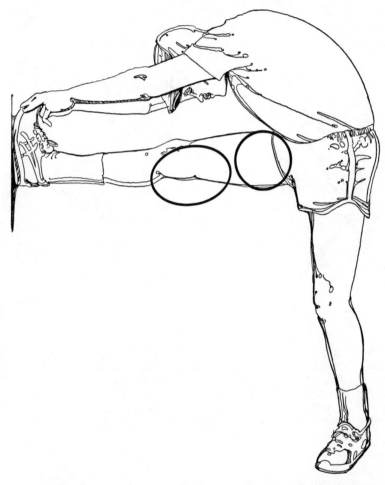

HAMSTRINGS AND GROIN. Choose a sturdy object waist high. Place back of heel on object while keeping leg straight. Raised leg must remain straight. Now bend forward slowly at the waist until a good stretch is felt in back of raised leg. Hold, relax, and then stretch further as it becomes easier to move head closer to raised foot. Stretch 30 seconds. Switch legs.

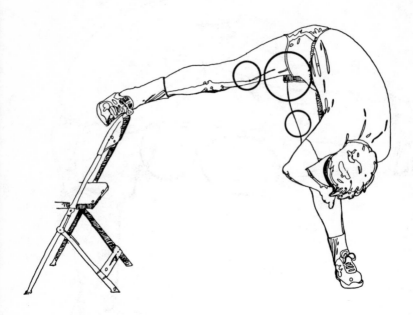

**HAMSTRINGS AND GROIN.** From the previous position, rotate foot on ground to the side keeping both legs straight, and bend at waist toward foot on ground. This exercise stretches the left and right hamstrings closer to buttock muscles. If you wish to stretch groin of raised leg, simply bend supporting knee as you reach toward ground, keeping raised leg straight. Stretch 30 seconds. Switch legs.

**SPINE AND WAISTLINE.** Stand with feet flat on ground about shoulder width apart. Keeping legs fairly straight, extend both arms overhead, grasp hands, and bend slowly to your left, and hold in a curved position for 30 seconds. Now bend to the right for 30 seconds. Keep back fairly upright during this exercise.

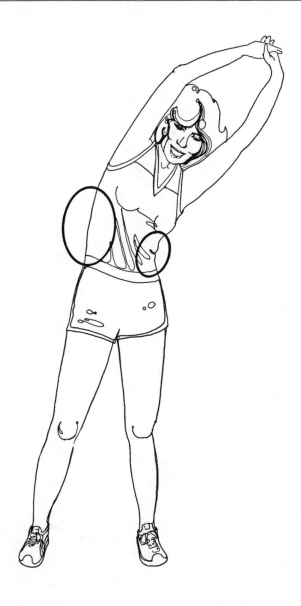

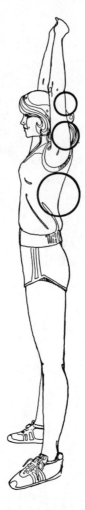

BACK, SHOULDERS, AND ARMS. With arms extended overhead and palms together, slowly stretch arms upward and backward. Keep elbows as straight as possible. Stretch for 10–15 seconds and repeat 2–3 times.

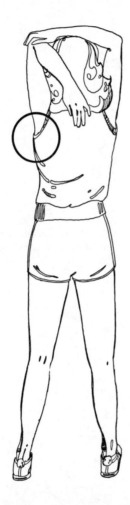

SHOULDERS AND TRICEP MUSCLE. With left elbow up behind head (left hand in center of back) grab left elbow with right hand and gently pull left elbow behind head. Don't apply a lot of force, just even pressure. Stretch for 10–15 seconds. Switch arms.

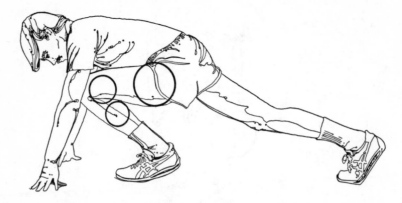

HIPS. Place left foot on ground, bend left knee, and place right leg straight behind. Keeping left foot fairly flat, lean forward without moving left knee position. Hip muscles will stretch. DON'T BOUNCE. Stretch 20–30 seconds. Switch legs.

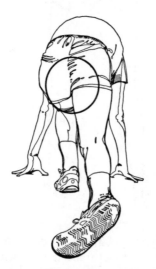

GROIN. Stay in previous position. Rotate right foot away from body. Seen from behind, the rotation would be away from other foot. Stretch 20–30 seconds. Switch legs.

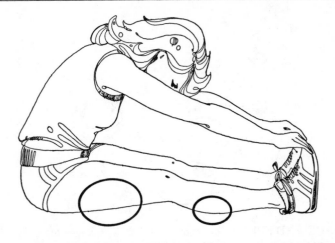

HAMSTRINGS AND CALF MUSCLES. Sit with legs stretched out straight ahead. Feet should be no more than 6–8 inches apart. Reach and touch toes. Stretch for 15–20 seconds touching toes, try to stretch and grab heels. You may also want to alternate hands (right hand grabbing left heel).

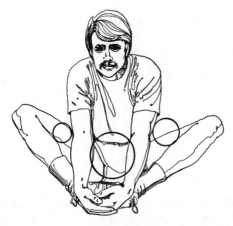

GROIN. Sit down, put the soles of feet together, and grab feet around ankles. *Gently* pull feet toward you until stretching is felt in groin. Stretch for 15–20 seconds.

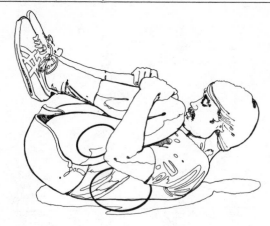

BACK AND SPINE. In a prone position, hold knees together with hands and pull knees up to chest keeping chin tucked against chest. *Gently* roll back spine and up on shoulders. Roll slowly 8–10 times.

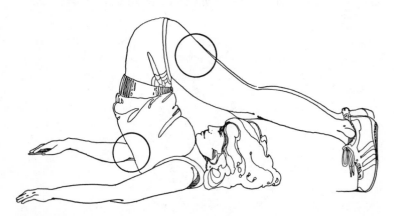

BACK. Slowly roll back on shoulders raising legs and feet overhead. *Do slowly* and keep hands under hips for support until back muscles are stretched. Then place arms flat on the ground. Extend legs fully and try to touch toes on the ground behind head. Stretch 20–30 seconds. Be careful not to choke off normal breathing pattern.

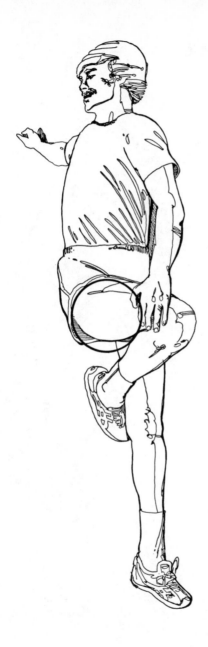

BACK AND SIDE OF HIP. Laying on back, bend right knee and roll to left until your knee crosses left leg and touches the floor. Keep both shoulders and head on the ground. Right arm should be extended straight out from the shoulder touching the ground. Left leg should be straight and flat on the floor. Now place left hand on right thigh (close to the knee) and press down. Turn head to the right. Stretch 20–30 seconds. Stretching is felt in back. Switch legs.

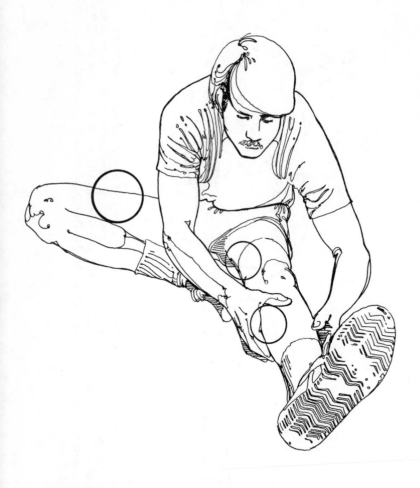

BACK OF LEG AND BACK. Start in a sitting position with left leg straight. (Note: Foot must be straight also.) Place the sole of the right foot flat against the inside left thigh, keeping the right knee on the floor. Bend forward at the waist toward the left foot until stretching is realized. Stretch 20–30 seconds. Switch legs.

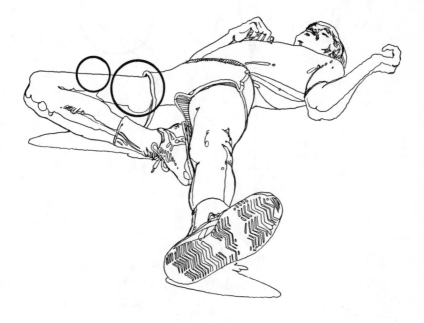

QUADRICEPS. Maintain previous sitting position. Lean *back* until stretching is felt in right thigh. Continue leaning back until head touches the ground. Stretch 20–30 seconds. Switch legs.

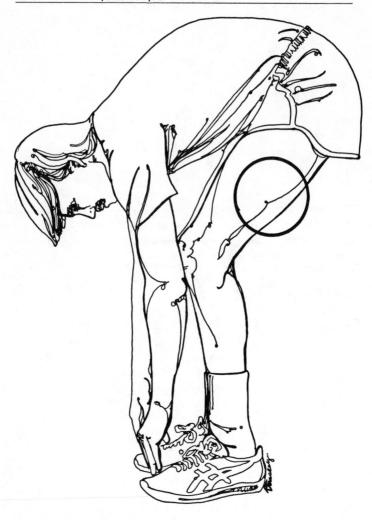

FINAL STRETCH FOR HAMSTRINGS. Stand erect. With knees bent, bend over and place hands on ground or under toes of shoes. Slowly straighten knees until you feel the hamstrings pull. Stretch 20–30 seconds.

## A THREE-PART STOMACH EXERCISE

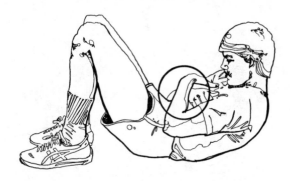

ABDOMINAL CURL. Start by lying on back with knees bent and feet flat on ground. Hands are crossed on chest. Tuck chin against chest and keep shoulders rounded. Curl up by bringing shoulder blades off the mat 6–8 inches. Keep shoulders rounded throughout the exercise. Lower back down to the starting position (usually about 3 inches from the ground). Concentrate on not jerking the head and keeping the exercise slow and steady. Try to repeat 10 times at first.

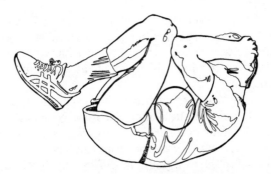

ELBOW-KNEE ABDOMINAL CURL. Still lying on back with knees bent, interlock fingers behind head and raise both feet off the ground. Now bring elbows toward knees with the help of the abdominal muscles. Aim elbows about two inches above the knees. Attempt to repeat 10 times. This is a difficult exercise and should be done slowly at first.

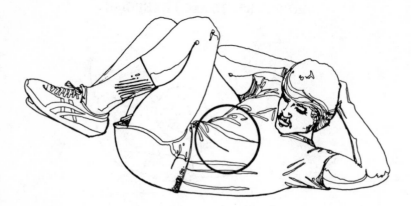

CROSS ELBOW--KNEE CURL.   Maintain the same position and touch the right elbow to the left thigh. Try not to jerk. Touch left elbow right thigh. Alternate elbow-thigh touching. Repeat 10 times.

the area is safe, and you wear clothing that can easily be seen by motorists. If you eat before jogging, allow three hours for digestion. Perhaps you could run directly after work, which would allow you to run in the daylight, at least during the summer months.

Another way to fit jogging into your life is by being alert to every opportunity for it. When you take your car in for servicing, why not run home from the garage and then back again later? You can run to and from the post office. Is it possible to run to and from your place of employment? Maybe you can take running clothes with you and run home from work. Walking is also exercise, so think about walking to the grocery store when you need only a few things like milk and bread which are not too heavy to carry.

When at work, attempt to walk up and down stairs rather

than taking the elevator. Walk to lunch rather than riding. Don't take short cuts by cutting corners—always walk farther than you have to (all exercise burns calories). Every calorie burned up walking or running will make your muscles more efficient metabolizers.

Certain circumstances put a strain on even the dedicated jogger. Business trips are one strain. When I go out of town I run early in the morning on the streets of the city I'm visiting. I jog around two square blocks. Many times you won't get to bed until late, but you will be glad you answered the ring of the alarm clock. Perhaps you could plan to run after the afternoon business meeting. Most meetings end at five o'clock, and usually dinners are not scheduled until seven. This allows you two hours for exercising and showering, and an opportunity to decrease your appetite before the evening meal. A jump rope can be put in your suitcase to be used in your hotel room if time is at such a premium that you can't run. You can also run in place to get your heart rate up to 80 percent of your maximum heart rate.

Do you get the point? *You must first of all decide you want to jog.* Then *make time* to jog. You really can find the time if you want, usually without sacrificing sleep or work performance.

*Soreness*

When you first start running your muscles will be sore. This should be expected. Sore legs are pretty much a part of the first stages of jogging, and an all-over stiffness will be noticed for several days when you first start to exercise. This will not harm you; it is your body's way of telling you that dormant muscle fibers are back to work.

A hot tub of water is sure to help the initial soreness. The soreness is a result of excess lactic acid build-up in the muscles and dissipates with time, usually 48-60 hours after exercise. The hot water causes vasodilation (opening of the blood vessels) and allows for faster evacuation of the lactic acid.

### Shoes

Think about what you are asking your feet to do as you go around the track or take off on your jog around the block! Each shoe lands on the ground approximately 800 times per mile. Since you have two feet this totals up to 1,600 times per mile. If you run three miles that is 4,800 times your shoes hit the ground. That is 4,800 jolts carried through your feet, to your ankles, knees, and hips. If you weigh 150 pounds that is a total impact of 360 tons during every three-mile workout.

*Tennis sneakers or basketball shoes just are not able to give your feet the necessary support* for 360 tons of impact over a three-mile course. Don't try to save money on shoes. Stay away from wholesale or second-rate shoes sold by chain stores.

Good shoes do the following things for your feet: 1) Because they fit right, they minimize blisters; 2) Because they are properly padded, they cushion shock on your feet, which is transmitted to the rest of your body; 3) Because they have a good stable heel, they keep lateral sway to a minimum and reduce wear and tear on your leg muscles. If you feel you must save money, do not save on footwear. Jogging is no fun if your feet are sore.

Good shoes are made by many manufacturers: Nike, Adidas, Tiger, Puma, New Balance, Converse, and Brooks, to name a few. Carefully check any shoe you are thinking about buying and don't take the word of the salesclerk to be the authority. Running shoes should fit snugly, not tightly, and should not pinch or cramp your toes nor let your foot slide forward, allowing your toes to jam against the toe of the shoe. Most running shoes fit one size larger than your street shoe size.

Running shoes should be flexible, especially at the ball of

the foot where it bends as you push off with each stride. If it doesn't flex with ease you will have to put needless effort on your legs. Before you buy a shoe I suggest you bend it. If it takes effort to bend the shoe then make another selection.

A stable heel is important. Look for one that is wide enough to give your foot good support when it hits the ground. Don't buy a running shoe with a narrow heel, especially if you are just starting to jog, as the narrow heel does not allow for good lateral support.

Take *time* to pick a good shoe. Don't worry about the weight of the shoe, as a few more ounces will not make much difference and will be worth any possible difference if you get a pleasant running experience. It is worth spending $25-$40 for good running shoes. That is cheaper than two visits to the doctor with sore feet or a chronic knee problem.

The care of shoes is really quite simple. If they get wet, let them dry slowly, away from heat, with shoe trees or crumpled paper stuffed in them. Heels that wear can be repaired with an electric glue gun if you care to add life to the heel and save replacement costs. If they start to stink, throw them in the washing machine on your day of rest.

### Orthotics

Dr. George Sheehan feels that many jogging pains can best be cured with special shoe inserts called *orthotics*. Dr. Sheehan says that "man was created to walk barefoot in the sand. When he stepped in the sand, the sand would create a perfect fit by conforming to the depressions and elevations on the bottom of his foot. Shoes cannot possibly fit your feet as well unless they are formed from a cast made of your foot." (59)

Why is the perfect fit on the bottom of your foot so important? When you jog, you land on your heel, come down on the outside part of your foot, and then roll your foot so that all your weight shifts to the inside part of your foot. This rolling from the outside part of your foot to the inside part of your foot is called pronation and is responsible for most injuries to joggers who run long distances. Good running shoes are designed to limit pronation.

Orthotics are expensive and should not be tried unless you are unable to get rid of foot, leg, or knee pain. Good shoes will usually give the foot, knees, and legs sufficient cushioning so that orthotics will not be necessary.

## Socks

Some runners prefer not to wear socks. I personally enjoy the cushion-like feel that a pair of cotton or wool socks give my feet. I find that cotton socks are cooler in the summer and don't allow my feet to become hot. Nylon can tear your skin or cause blisters and should be avoided. Tennis anklers, made of cotton, are very comfortable on hot days. You might try running without socks to see if it is to your liking. Some runners prefer the feel of having their feet in direct contact with their shoes.

## Shorts

Nylon shorts which have a split up the side are best for jogging. They allow room for contraction of the thigh muscles. Nylon is light and cool for summer days and will dry quickly after getting wet. Cotton shorts absorb moisture and feel heavy if you are sweating a great deal.

## Long Pants

In the winter you may want to wear long john underwear to shield you against the bitter cold. The pants of a jogging suit that are not too loose (allowing for loss of heat) can be worn over the long john underwear. Some joggers like leotard pants worn under cotton shorts if it is not too cold. I personally don't like sweat pants on a cold, snowy day because they get wet and seem to weigh a ton. Close fitting pants keep body heat in and thus help keep your legs warm during exercise.

*Support*

For men, a jock strap is good to wear on a hot day because it minimizes chapping in the groin area. However, on a cool day, I prefer to use jockey shorts to give me the necessary support. Again, this is an area where you will want to experiment. A narrow waistband on a jock will prevent curling, which can cause the material to cut into your side.

Running bras are available for women which help hold the breasts more firmly than regular bras. Regular bras sometimes do not provide sufficient support. Ask at your local running shop or at better-stocked department stores.

*Shirts*

In the summer, most men prefer to run without a shirt, or at most wear a tank-top type shirt. Loosely woven, net type material allows for the escape of body heat during your summer runs. Women can also wear tank-top shirts which are cooler than T-shirts.

As the temperature gets cooler, first put on a T-shirt. If you are still cold, try a long-sleeved T-shirt; then add a sweatshirt, and finally go to a light nylon jacket, which holds body heat in and does not allow the wind to get through as you jog.

*Gloves*

Leather ski gloves are part of my winter exercise program. For some reason, my hands get cold quickly, even on mildly cold days. Therefore, leather ski gloves help me very much. Most people find, however, that their hands sweat in ski gloves and wearing wool gloves or mittens is more comfortable. Mittens are warmer since your fingers are in direct contact with each other and retain heat. Famous marathoner Bill Rodgers likes to wear garden gloves. (Bill won the 1978 Boston Marathon wearing a pair of garden gloves.) Gardening gloves are quite inexpensive and will wash easily if dirty.

## Hats

Forty percent of your body heat escapes from your head, so wear a hat in the winter. On cold days you will see joggers wearing a sweatshirt hood over their sweating head. I personally like a simple wool ski hat that keeps my ears warm. A full ski mask can be worn on really cold days.

On warm days, especially at fun runs, plain visors that golfers sometimes wear are often seen. I personally get along nicely with my sweatband and don't use a visor. Sunglasses can be worn on bright, sunny days to shield your eyes. Find what suits you best.

## Sweatbands

I personally like a sweatband around my forehead because it keeps sweat out of my eyes. Without a sweatband I am constantly rubbing sweat from my eyes, which irritates the skin. Try a sweatband; you may or may not like it. I also like to run without a T-shirt in the summer, but some people feel that the sweat running down their backs gets their jogging shorts too wet. Try different things. You will learn what works best for you!

## Rubberized Suits

Rubberized suits should never be used to lose weight. Wrestlers often use such suits to help them lose weight to make a certain weight class. Is it weight loss if I sweat two pounds of perspiration from my body and keep it off only until I drink a glass of fluid or eat? My dehydrated body needs the water from the food and the two pounds are back where they were before I started exercising. Rubber suits are useless in weight loss and prevent the body from getting rid of excess heat from normal exercise. Your body needs to cool off by perspiring. Rubber suits can easily cause heat exhaustion.

*Timing*

It is better to run a certain amount of time rather than concentrating on distance. A regular wristwatch gives the time accurately within 30-40 seconds. As you improve your health your speed will automatically increase. Perhaps when you notice you are running faster you will want to get a stopwatch, which is easier to read and more accurate. Stopwatches are not necessary to good health, but they help satisfy our egos. Improvement in time or distance makes us set new goals. With each new goal comes a desire to accomplish that goal and go on to the next plateau.

A watch is useful when running an unfamiliar course or when you are on business trips or vacations. With a watch you will have some idea as to how far you've gone, and when you are to the half-way point and need to start back to your motel.

Many wristwatches today are so sophisticated that they are stopwatches, timers, gauge knots per minute, and accomplish everything but run for you. You know what your needs are, so decide whether your normal wristwatch will suffice. For at least the first two years after starting an exercise program, most everyone should not use anything but a wristwatch, as *time spent doing* the exercise is more important than the *speed of doing* the exercise.

*Choose a Reasonable Goal*

A new exercise program should be done safely, slowly, and progressively. Listed in the back of Dr. Cooper's book, *The Aerobic Way*, is a point system for the different exercises. (19) I recommend a time period rather than a point system, but both are based on the same foundation. I feel you should not be concerned with the distance traveled but with the amount of *time spent exercising and expending energy*. For the novice runner a suggested schedule is listed below. Tuesday and Thursday vary with other days in order to add variety to the exercise schedule.

| | |
|---|---|
| Monday, Wednesday, Friday | 8 minutes after warm-up period |
| Tuesday and Thursday | 12 minutes after warm-up period |
| Saturday | 15 minutes after warm-up period |
| Sunday | REST (Your muscles need one day's rest per week to replenish the glycogen used up with six days of exercise.) |

As stated earlier, if your present health condition is such that fast walking gets your heat rate up to 80 percent MHR, you should do warm-up exercises and then walk briskly for eight minutes. The above schedule should be followed until you can do it comfortably without being overly tired most of the day after exercising. It is normal to be comfortably tired during the first two weeks of an aerobic schedule. Usually two to three weeks is sufficient breaking in time for a new running schedule.

After the third or fourth week the following schedule is recommended for a second goal.

| | |
|---|---|
| Monday, Wednesday, Friday | 10 minutes after warm-up period |
| Tuesday and Thursday | 15 minutes after warm-up period |
| Saturday | 20 minutes after warm-up period |
| Sunday | REST |

Of course, it is understood that the above time periods are continuous jogging and not jogging and walking combined. If you must walk part of the time, you are not ready to advance to the next increased time schedule.

The ultimate goal is to be able to jog using 80 percent of maximal heart rate for the following periods of time. This is a long-range goal and may take up to three to four years to accomplish. It is suggested that you increase each day only two minutes per week. It is better to take it slowly and not get discouraged. The ultimate goal:

| | |
|---|---|
| Monday, Wednesday, Friday | 36 minutes after warm-up period |
| Tuesday and Thursday | 45 minutes after warm-up period |
| Saturday | 60 minutes after warm-up period |
| Sunday | REST |

This schedule was my goal to achieve. It is not necessary for you ever to achieve this ultimate. You can become healthy by attaining goals of 30-40 minutes per day. Use your own judgment in setting your jogging goals. After you are fit, exercise of 15-20 minutes per day will maintain your fitness.

However, it seems to me that the schedule above is within the reach of most anyone who wants to improve the temple that God has loaned him. Running at the nine-minute pace per mile is in reach of most anyone within three years of beginning as a jogger, if weight is proper. This means running four miles on Monday, Wednesday, Friday; five miles on Tuesday and Thursday; and six and one-half miles on Saturday. Remember, this is a goal to strive for and not a schedule that should be attempted until you have been *jogging for years* and are in good health.

How can you monitor your performance? Are you pushing it too hard? The immediate signs of overexertion to look for *during* exercise are pain in the chest; difficulty in breathing, such as gasping or gulping for air; light-headedness; feeling that your muscle control lacks coordination; and nausea. If you experience any of the above symptoms during exercise, slow down or stop immediately until the symptoms leave. If the chest pain persists, see a physician immediately.

Signs of exercising too hard often express themselves in the form of fatigue. This usually manifests itself by excessive drowsiness in the late afternoon or early evening. Irritability over little pressures is also a sign of being over-exercised.

*Cooling Down After Exercise*

A person will run a horse in a race and then spend time walking and rubbing the animal down afterward, so the horse can cool down properly. However, that same animal-loving individual will run for 25 minutes, stop immediately, and sit down to rest. Take at least 5-10 minutes to cool down to avoid nausea and cramps. The muscles have been asking the heart to supply excess blood while exercising. After completion of the exercise the heart needs an adjustment period to stop pushing excess blood to the muscles.

It is also recommended that you do not complete a strenuous exercise and step into a sauna (dry heat), steam bath (wet heat), or a hot shower. Your heart is still in need of excess blood, and when you step into a sauna the blood goes to the capillaries of the skin surface to cool your body instead of to the heart.

Think about walking at least five minutes after a jogging exercise. Walk faster at the start of the slowdown and taper to a normal walking pace at the end of the slowdown period.

After walking you should do stretching exercises again. As we run our muscles become short and thick. After jogging you will find you are actually stiffer than before you jogged. *Please* stretch the hamstring, calf, and back muscles. Also stretch the Achilles tendon. Stretching is just as important *after* exercise as *before* exercise. (Refer to the stretching exercises described earlier in this chapter.)

It has already been mentioned that cold drinks are not advised immediately after strenuous exercise. Drink cool to slightly above room temperature water immediately after exercising if you feel you need liquid. The most ideal situation is to cool down, take a shower, and then drink liquid after your body has adjusted.

*Check Your Recovery Pulse*

*Immediately* after completing your jogging exercise, it is important to take your carotid pulse. The carotid artery is found on the side of the neck just under the angle of the jaw. Use the fingertips rather than your thumb, and only one hand. If both hands are used it is possible to become light-headed or pass out. The carotid artery is very easy to find after exercising because it is engorged with precious blood needed by your heart, muscles, and brain cells.

The pulse should be taken immediately after stopping the exercise because the heart rate usually slows down rapidly.

It is easy to take your pulse for *six seconds* and then multiply it by a factor of ten to get your beats per minute rate.

Example: 14 beats in 6 seconds × factor 10 = 140 beats per minute.

In this example 80 percent of the maximal heart rate is 140 beats per minute. After walking for one minute the heart rate should have dropped 25 to 40 points in a well-conditioned heart. In five minutes the rate should have dropped 40 to 50 points. If your heart rate is still 120 after five minutes, it is advisable to seek advice from your physician.

CAUTION. Take your pulse *immediately* after exercise. If you wait 10 seconds your heart rate could drop 15 to 20 beats.

## God's Guidelines

God tells us in Proverbs 3:1,2, "My son, do not forget my teaching, but let your heart keep my commandments; For length of days and years of life, and peace they will add to you." God wants us to have increased days—long life—and for those days to be healthy.

Saint John said, "Beloved, I pray that in all respects you may prosper and be *in good health*, just as your soul prospers" (3 John 2, italics mine).

God wants us to be healthy, and we can be healthy, if we use the preceding guidelines for our future health and happiness. Keep a personal chart of how many minutes you run each day. This is usually best kept on your monthly calendar. Be honest with yourself as you record your progress. Remember, God expects you to put forth the effort to get His temple healthy.

Your doctor can tell you that you *appear* to be in fairly good shape, but if you don't *feel healthy*, what difference does it make what your doctor tells you? From a physical, as well as from a mental and spiritual standpoint, fitness obtained from aerobic exercise will put more energy into you, more years into your life, and most importantly, more life into your remaining years. Can you afford not to exercise?

# CHAPTER 8

## Braving the Elements

Let me be painfully honest for a moment—and intensely personal. Sometimes God uses unusual situations to gain our attention. For me, it was a rude awakening not to overdo things on a very hot day.

Humidity together with heat is the absolute worst combination possible for a jogger. The heat causes your body temperature to increase and the humidity, if high enough, does not allow the sweat which is produced to evaporate properly.

I and five of my jogging partners ran a 10,000 meter (6.2 miles) fun run July 22, 1978, in Delaware, Ohio. The race started at 10 A.M., with the temperature at 86°F and the humidity at 93 percent. Since this was a fun run and many of us run together each morning, I suggested we take our time and just have a goal of finishing the race. I should have listened to my own advice.

Two of us had been running six miles on Mondays, Wednesdays, and Fridays, so the 10,000 meter distance was not itself a problem. The problem arose when I ran the first mile in 7.08 minutes. (We jog comfortably at a pace of 8.15 minutes per mile.) After the first mile I slowed my pace to the 8-minute rate and rounded the three-mile mark at 23.01 minutes. The temperature outdoors was now at 95°F, unbeknown to me.

My time was 38.31 at the five-mile mark. At this time and pace of the fun run, I was very hot and tired but not weary.

Enter the old high school Heller ego. I decided to speed up

to catch my younger friend who was about 50 yards ahead of me. When we got to within 400 yards of the finish line, I had closed within 20 yards of my friend. My brain told my legs to go as fast as they could, and I started sprinting. The last 300 yards of the race are foggy in my mind, because an abrupt personal encounter with the track is the last I remember of the race. I passed out on *terra firma* because of the combination of heat and humidity, sprinkled with the "Heller dumbs."

I wish that was the end of the story. Two runners who had finished the race helped me to my feet. I was gasping frantically for air as my lungs begged for oxygen. They carried me to shade underneath the stadium bleachers.

In about five minutes my other running partners came over to help. By this time, my body temperature had increased and I had stopped sweating altogether. It was hard to breathe because I was experiencing high "oxygen debt." Realizing that such heat exhaustion can cause tremendously high body temperature, I asked my friends to carry me to the middle of the football field where a water hose was running.

After being doused with water, I could feel my body temperature decrease, but it was becoming more difficult for me to breathe. As a matter of fact, *I was having a great deal of difficulty breathing.* My feet and hands began to tingle and then went numb. The color slowly left my skin, changing from tan to a pale white, and then my toenails and fingernails took on a bluish tint. I am told I became unconscious and quit breathing for a short period of time, until an emergency squadsman who had arrived on the scene leaned over me and screamed into my ear, "Start breathing!" He told me to breathe hard by pushing against his hand, which he was holding on my stomach. This pressure made me push my stomach out and thus force my diaphragm down, filling up my lungs with air.

*Please understand!* I was not fat or out of shape. I had

played football in high school at 162 pounds, but I only weighed 149 pounds the morning of the Delaware Fun Run. I was jogging 35 miles per week with at least three days of six-mile jogs. *I tried to do too much, too hard,* considering the heat and humidity. Heat and humidity combine to form a trap with steel jaws that can snap on anyone, even the conditioned athlete.

Run in the early morning hours when it is cool. Avoid the midday summer heat. Above all, don't run when there is a combination of high humidity and high temperature.

## Heat Exhaustion or Heatstroke?

We must consider heat exhaustion and heatstroke together, because it is most important in first aid to be able to distinguish between them. Heat exhaustion needs care, but it is usually not life-threatening. Heatstroke is rare, but it is definitely life-threatening and calls for fast action.

In both conditions the victim collapses. In heat exhaustion, the skin is pale, cool, and moist, and body temperature is about normal. But in heatstroke, the person's skin is reddened, fiery hot to the touch, and dry; his temperature may be 106°F or more. With either condition the victim will be disoriented at best and probably unconscious, especially with heatstroke.

Early treatment of heat exhaustion should include the following steps: Move the victim to a cool spot and try to get him to drink salty liquid. Also, remove his clothing and cool him off by bathing him with cloths soaked in cool water or alcohol. Usually the person feels better immediately, but if he seems fatigued, is elderly, or has a chronic disease, he should see a doctor. In any case, he should take it very easy for two or three days, meanwhile salting his food heavily.

If the person is obviously feverish, it is probably heatstroke, and minutes count. You must get his temperature started down or he is in trouble. Call for an ambulance, strip off his clothes, and start cooling with whatever means you can find. A bath in a tub of cold water and ice is ideal, but a massage with ice cubes or ice packs is more likely to be practicable. Rub the victim's arms, legs, and especially the stomach with handfuls of ice. The patient should be rushed to a hospital emergency room as soon as possible, so professionals can take over.

Heatstroke and heat exhaustion are avoidable with common sense. HEAT plus HUMIDITY set the stage for both problems. Humidity is more damaging than heat.

The National Joggers Association recommends that long distance races "should not be conducted when the wet bulb temperature-globe temperature exceeds 82.4°F." (49) Dr. David Costill, author of a special paper sponsored by the American College of Sports Medicine on the dangers of overheating in runners during the summer months, states that "a hot day of 90 degrees with 40 percent humidity is much better than a mild day of 60 degrees with 90 percent humidity for long distance running." Dr. Costill, himself a jogger and the director of the Human Performance Laboratory at Ball State University in Muncie, Indiana, insists that "strong warnings should be issued every spring to the joggers on the hazards of heatstroke and heat exhaustion." (21)

### Running at Night

If you run at night, do not wear dark clothing. The steel of an automobile is much harder than a jogger's flesh!

In cool weather, if your nylon windbreaker is dark, put a white T-shirt on over it. You also can place strips of reflective tape on your clothes or shoes to help oncoming motorists see you. If possible run on a not-so-well-traveled road.

Whatever you wear, run facing oncoming traffic so you are able to see the headlights coming at you. Don't look directly into the beam of the headlights, as this will cause you to see spots and very much limit your vision. Try to look ahead, memorizing the terrain of your next few steps, and then look away, catching only the edge of the headlights in your line of vision.

If a neighborhood track is open, this is the ideal place to run when it is dark. Your eyes will adapt quickly and you will be able to see the stripes on the track. Most nights the moon sheds enough light to enable you to see quite well.

## Heat

Exercising in hot weather for an extended period of time causes you to sweat and lose body fluid. This fluid loss should be replaced after exercising to avoid hypertension. Dehydration can cause headaches, excess fatigue, or a general lack of energy.

It is suggested that after exercising you avoid very cold drinks, as they often cause stomach pains and irregularity of heart rhythm. (People with past heart disease should *never* drink cold water directly after exercising.)

Excess sweating also causes a loss of electrolytes, which can be replaced by drinking ERG or Gatorade. Use of salt at mealtimes also helps retain blood electrolytes. ERG and Gatorade are high in sugar content and should be limited in quantity.

Our sweat glands wet our body enough to keep body temperature within its proper range in most circumstances. If the body's thermoregulatory mechanism can't keep the temperature low enough, heat cramps, heat exhaustion, or heatstroke is the result.

On hot days it is advisable to slow your pace. Unless you are running at the hottest time of the day, you should be able to run the predetermined amount of time but at a *slower pace.* If you find you are getting dizzy or that the heat is "getting" to you, slow down or walk until you feel like continuing. If you do not feel like jogging anymore, just walk back to your starting point.

Heat, especially temperatures above 85-90 degrees, de-serves our consideration. Only one fourth of the energy we produce is converted to movement; the other 75 percent is converted into heat. If your body is not able to rid itself of the heat, you will become overheated, just like a car with a hot radiator. Dehydration is like our car radiator boiling over. We lose valuable body fluid plus electrolytes, such as sodium chloride, magnesium, and potassium, a loss which can inter-fere with muscle contraction. *Don't allow your radiator to lose valuable fluid.*

## Cold

If you run outdoors during the colder months, it is sug-gested that you wear warm clothing (long johns if necessary) to keep warm. A paper-thin nylon windbreaker with a sweatshirt underneath, as well as a cap over your ears, will prevent valuable body heat loss during exercise. When running at below zero temperatures, use a surgical mask or knitted ski mask over the mouth and nose to warm up the air before it enters the lung tissue. Many drugstores sell masks especially for people with past heart disease who want to shovel snow during cold weather. These masks work nicely for the cold weather jogger. Loose-fitting mittens keep your hands warmer than gloves that fit snugly on the hands.

However, it is important during cold weather that you not overdress. Excess clothes make you work harder and cause you to perspire excessively. Wear only enough clothes to keep warm, allowing for evaporation of perspiration. During cool or not really cold weather, it is recommended that you wear several layers of light clothing. Peel off clothing as your body gets warmer from the exercise.

Because running is such an individual matter, what works for 99 percent of the joggers may not work for you. If something seems sensible, like wearing a big, heavy coat that keeps you warm, try it. If it doesn't work, or doesn't work as well as you would like, try something else.

## Rain

Running in the rain is a new experience that can be enjoyed by those willing to take a chance and try something different. There is such a "neat" feeling about drops of rain hitting you in the face and giving you a soothing feeling as you jog. Wanda, my wife, thought I was crazy to run in the rain until she tried it.

After running in the rain your body will be refreshed and will feel even "wetter" in the shower. Your mental image of yourself will increase five notches for having done something that others (except avid runners) usually avoid. Try it—you'll like it.

Rain is enjoyable to run in, but *lightning should be avoided altogether*. Lightning is dangerous and extremely unpredictable. Do not run if lightning can be seen or heard.

## Snow

Running when it is snowing, if you are dressed properly, can give you the same "high" as running in the rain. Due to your body temperature, the snow melts as it lands on your face and leaves it cool but not cold. Wind combined with snow is what makes your face feel cold. Don't avoid the benefits of jogging because of snow. You will be glad you did it, and your temple will stay healthy during the winter months.

## Wind

Whether during the summer or the winter, winds of more than 8-10 miles per hour are a decided resistance to your running. Running into a wind will slow you down, but not as much as you might think. Put your head down, lean into it, and make the best of it. That same wind is a pleasure when it is at your back, pushing you along.

Wind only becomes a problem in very cold temperatures. This is because of the wind-chill factor. For example, at +10°F a 10 mph wind gives a chill factor of −9°F, and a 20 mph wind gives a chill factor of −25°F. So, during cold, windy weather try to run where there is as much shelter from the wind as possible. Better still, invest in a three-month membership at the YMCA or YWCA.

### Ice

Avoid running on ice, as it is easy to fall and the injuries can be serious. If possible, run later in the day to allow the sun to melt ice on the roads. Again, an indoor track is the best solution to this problem.

### Sand

When you go on vacation and are anxious to get to the beach to jog, *be careful!* Wear your regular running shoes. If you run without shoes, your feet, not being accustomed to the sand, will become raw without your noticing it until the next day. Sand is very abrasive and will wear the epithelial layer off the soles of your feet. It is better to run in your shoes and then enjoy walking on the beach in your bare feet after your run.

### Fog

Running in fog is much like running in the dark, except that you can usually see the road ahead. Remember that motorists driving in the fog are at more of a handicap than the runner: They aren't looking for you, so you must watch for them. Don't wear gray clothing in the fog, as you will blend into the background and be invisible to the motorist. Red, yellow, and orange are good colors to wear in the fog.

### Dogs

If you run regularly, you will undoubtedly come face to face with an angry dog. Every serious jogger has a war story to tell about how he or she handled a canine guerilla.

Most dog owners deeply believe their dog is incapable of doing wrong; plus their dog has his rights! If a dog runs at you, even though you are on the other side of the street, most dog owners will look on and feel their dog has a right to run at you. In short, you can expect little sympathy from dog owners.

Most dogs are assiduous defenders of turf. They quickly learn what are their territorial limits and they defend those borders. If a passing jogger doesn't appear to threaten these borders, a harmless warning bark is usually the only result. Therefore, you might want to cross the street and avoid the dog's territory.

You may have to bluff an approaching dog. Pick up a rock or stick and act like you are throwing it at the dog. This approach usually makes the dog think twice about biting at your heels.

Hopefully a stern approach—saying "No!" or "Stop!"— will suffice in letting the dog know you are willing to defend yourself. But above all, *don't act afraid*. Dogs are adept at recognizing fear and thus become more aggressive.

Some runners are noted for carrying a bottle of ammonia water and squirting it at the dog. This teaches the dog you mean business and plan to run this path in the future. Ammonia will burn the eyes of the dog, but he will get over it.

## Identification Tags or Bracelets

Try to picture a runner jogging along a sunny road on a beautiful fall day. The runner has just started to sweat and get that good feeling.

Suddenly a pain is felt in the chest and dizziness overcomes equilibrium. The runner falls to the side of the road, unconscious. An emergency vehicle is summoned, and the runner is taken to the nearest local hospital. No identification can be found on the runner. This could happen to you or anyone.

Identification bracelets or identification shoe tags should

be worn anytime you jog. Even if you jog a regularly traveled path, an accident may occur and you may not be recognized. It is difficult for policemen to identify a jogger without proper means.

The identification should include your name, address, home and business telephone numbers, name of person to be notified in an emergency, and any vital medical information. When jogging in another city, you should carry your hotel room key with you for identification purposes.

All of us think an accident could not happen to us—only to the other person. But what if you fall with a sprained ankle or get hit with a bicycle—or worse, an automobile? If you are conscious you can explain the necessary personal information to medical authorities. If you are unconscious an identification tag might save your life, and make it easier for others to contact your closest relative.

# CHAPTER 9

## The 25 Most-Often-Asked Questions About Exercise

The following are questions often asked by individuals starting an exercise program.

1. *What about walking?*

Dr. L. L. Lamb, editor of the *Health Letter*, states:

A number of different investigations have established the value of simple walking in improving the overall health. One of the most important things that walking does is to use calories. It helps in preventing and controlling obesity. A 150-pound individual walking at a speed of three miles an hour will utilize approximately 60 calories per mile more than he would if he were resting. For such an individual to walk one hour a day, or three miles, would mean that he would use 180 additional calories a day as a result of his exercise. A single day's walking will not produce any appreciable decrease in fat deposits in the body, but if such an individual walks an hour a day for one year, he will use the same number of calories present in 19 pounds of fat provided, of course, he doesn't increase his calorie intake enough to cancel out the beneficial effects of the exercise on calorie control. (46)

Elderly people should be encouraged to walk up to a mile before taking a taxi. Also, walking up and down flights of stairs rather than riding elevators or escalators is beneficial.

2. *What about riding a stationary bicycle?*

Some people enjoy using a stationary bicycle which, like running in place, has the advantage of being an exercise that can be done indoors. (I have found that you can read your Bible while riding a stationary bicycle on snowy days when jogging is impractical.) Most stationary bicycles have a means of adjusting the tension on the wheel so that the amount of work required can gradually be increased.

The basic principles for jogging also apply to bicycling whether on stationary or ordinary bicycles: Start at a low level and gradually increase the tension or speed, thus avoiding overexertion at peak levels of exercising. But *do increase the tension* every so often as you progress in strength from doing the exercise.

### 3. *How many calories does exercise burn up?*

Advocates against exercising say that you don't burn up enough calories to warrant the effort. It has been estimated (Cooper [19] and Bailey [9]) that if Frank Shorter, an Olympic marathoner, runs a five and one-half minutes per mile pace, he burns up 10-11 calories per minute. An individual jogging a mile in nine or ten minutes burns up approximately nine calories per minute.

At that rate, an individual will burn 100 calories per mile. If he jogs two miles in 20 minutes, that only equals 200 calories expended, which is a little more than a glass of milk or two pieces of white bread.

If that were the conclusion of the matter, I would agree that is a lot of effort for only 200 calories. However, after exercising for 20 minutes our blood vessels are dilated, our heart works harder, and our muscles continue to demand glucose for energy. For a period of four to six hours after exercise, our bodies use up more calories just to maintain a normal metabolism rate. The "high" or "good feeling" we experience after exercise is at the price of burning up more calories at rest than if we had not exercised.

The fit person continues to burn calories at a higher rate

after exercise than before exercise. So ladies, jog in the morning. Then think how many more calories you are using up doing the dishes today than yesterday when you didn't have time to jog.

4. *How do I combat the boredom and monotony of exercising?*

Exercise is work, but a pleasant work, and such a reward for the effort. The good feeling, mentally and physically, we receive from exercise is so beneficial that most runners feel the end result outweighs the monotony.

Boredom can be overcome by running with someone or joining a group that has regular planned runs. Carrying on a conversation while jogging with a friend makes time fly and the distance seem shorter.

Tom and Jan Bernard run each day with Wanda and me. Tom and I run at our pace, discussing situations or problems that we encounter at work.

Since Tom is president of a company and is familiar with management problems, he is of great assistance to my small dental office problems. Jan and Wanda run at their pace and talk about their own situations and problems. Since we all jog on a quarter-mile track, Tom and I chat with the ladies, too, as we go by at a slightly faster pace.

This brings up the question of the pace for people jogging together. Say one is in better shape or has been jogging longer than his partner. How do you handle that situation? What works best is for the faster runner to go at the slower runner's pace until the latter is finished. Then, the faster runner can go one or two additional laps at a quicker pace.

Another friend, Tom Driskell, finds that he is more comfortable running with Tom and me at our pace for 10 minutes and then dropping back to a more relaxed pace.

As you can see, there are many solutions to the problem of

boredom. Friends who run with you are some of the greatest friends with whom you will ever be associated. You are all getting healthier and enjoying friendship, day by day.

Since the members of our group live close to each other, we each enjoy the added benefit of overcoming laziness. We take turns driving to the track. If Tom drove yesterday, it is my turn to drive today. Even if I would like to stay in bed because I had a late meeting the night before, I feel very uncomfortable calling Tom at 5:30 A.M. to tell him Wanda and I have decided to "sack-in" on our morning to drive. How many times each one of us has said, "If it weren't for you coming to pick me up this morning (or the fact that it was my turn to drive), I would have gone back to bed."

Look around. There may be a jogging individual or group in your neighborhood or apartment complex. They would love to have you join them. They will not be boring!

When I must jog by myself, I have learned to be content with my own thoughts. Perhaps the following will give you an idea how to use the time alone.

After running a couple of warm-up laps I settle into my normal pace and proceed to run a predetermined amount of time. There are five members in my family, including myself. I pray for one person for one lap and then pick another member to pray for while running the next lap.

When running on a bike trail or road, I pick out an object in the distance, such as a telephone pole or tree, and pray for a certain family member until I jog to that landmark. Then I pick another object in the distance and select another family member to pray for until I reach the next object.

5. *Will I make a fool of myself if I jog?*

There are 20-25 million runners in the United States, of which 25,000 actually run 26-mile marathons. In Hawaii, for example, recovered heart attack patients run the Honolulu

Marathon wearing black shirts with large, red, broken hearts stitched on them.

Try to remember there are probably hundreds of people in your area who jog, not at the same hour perhaps, but on the same path or road that you use. Most people admire what you are doing. Also keep in mind that the people we feel are watching are so wrapped up in their own thoughts that a jogger hardly registers in their brain. The jogger just becomes part of the scenery.

Most people take to jogging like ducks take to water. It is not something we must learn to do, like tennis or golf, because we did it as a child. We must just do it now with perhaps a lot of extra weight.

Don't be ashamed of working to get yourself back into shape. And should kids in passing cars make sarcastic remarks, remember those comments are usually intended to impress the passengers in the car, not to nail the individual who received them.

### 5. Should I hold my arms a certain way while jogging?

Let your arms swing comfortably at your side, parallel to your body movement. Try to let them relax. They should neither flop in front of your chest nor be held rigid. Most runners hold their arms bent at the elbow roughly at right angles to the body. Perhaps the best advice is to forget about how you hold them and run with your arms in a position that is comfortable for you.

### 7. Should I breathe a certain way while jogging?

Many joggers ask, "How should I breathe while jogging?" or "Should I breathe with my mouth open?"

Some time ago a theory got started that runners should breathe in through the nose and out through the mouth.

Jogging calls for a lot of air to satisfy the body's need for oxygen. You won't last long breathing in only through your nose.

Breathing should be relaxed, through the mouth and nose, and it should follow "belly breathing" principles. Most of us breathe backwards. We tend to suck our stomachs in and breathe from the chest. With proper abdominal breathing the belly expands as you breathe in and flattens as you breathe out. The expansion of the abdomen indicates that the diaphragm is fully lowered, inflating the lungs completely and allowing a more efficient intake of oxygen. Improper breathing can also cause a "side stitch" or side cramp.

Don't get hung up on proper breathing. Just practice breathing deeply through your stomach rather than your chest. It is not hard to do and will become a natural part of your running after a short period of time.

8. *Is there a correlation between jogging and mental outlook?*

Is it not impossible to separate the mental and the physical? If your stomach hurts it is hard for you to concentrate on your daily devotions. The reverse is also true: If your stomach feels fine it is much easier for you to read the Bible or experience mental awareness in general.

If you jog and experience a new physical high from running through the park, your mental outlook is going to be better because you feel good.

Improved cardiovascular fitness through exercise, diet, weight control, and proper rest has a definite direct affect on the brain. The increased blood flow that is directed to our muscles to supply needed oxygen also goes to our brain and supplies the brain cells with oxygen and blood glucose, which keeps us thinking more clearly. If your brain has more oxygen and glucose, you are more wide awake and better able to handle stressful situations.

A study was done at a medical college trying to find the effect of exercise on helping students to think more efficiently. Fifty percent of the class was required to run one mile each day just before the class started. At the end of the quarter, those students who exercised got 16 percent higher grades than those students who stayed with their normal routine.

The next quarter the class reversed the experiment. Those who did not run the first quarter were now expected to run one mile before the class. The results were similar.

The conclusion drawn from the experiment was that due to the increased blood oxygen levels from exercise, the brain was more alert and able to function more efficiently. (20) Jim Fixx says, "Most people who exercise regularly after the age of 30 feel they would prefer to run in the morning before a 'pressure day,' as they are able to handle the pressure differently after exercise." (24)

People who are asked why they keep jogging after achieving a desired weight often reply, "It makes me feel so good, even after I stop exercising." I think it is your brain as well as your physical body that is experiencing that good feeling.

## 9. What are the psychological effects of exercise?

Is your mind playing tricks on you by telling you that you feel better than you actually do? If my mind tells me that I feel great even though my body is tired after a long day at the office, all I can say is, "Thank God." Is not happiness achieved when we feel great or have achieved a predetermined goal?

Few psychological frontiers are more intriguing than the changes that occur in your mind as a result of running. Some of these feelings are a sense of increased mental awareness and concentration, increased willpower, increased ability to work harder during fatigue, relief of tension, and the acceptance of pain. It is a good mental feeling to be successful, whether it be closing a sale or running your first 10-minute mile!

One thing that almost always happens with exercise is that your sense of self-worth increases, as you compare yourself to yesterday's standards. You accept yourself a little better when you run. At your own speed you can go where you want and think your own thoughts.

Most runners find they have considerably more energy than non-runners. This contributes to a feeling of greater control over their lives. Vaughan Thomas, in *Science and Sport*, observed that "we spend much of our lives dominated by others, such as sergeants in the Army, bosses, mothers-in-law, or leaders, who tell us what we will do and what we are not allowed to do. As a result, our need for self-assertion is constantly being pushed out of the way. Jogging gives us a socially acceptable way of asserting ourselves, of being as competitive, with ourselves or with others, as we want to be." (62)

If you jog at night you can get away from the television set for a period of time. In my opinion television is basically useless unless it is used for educational purposes. So instead of watching television, spend that time exercising your body.

### 10. *Do children need to exercise?*

Most children are very active and burn up their caloric intake rapidly up to age 10. Many children after age 10 start to put on weight because of eating more (usually junk food) calories than what their bodies burn up during activity.

Some children over 10 need to be encouraged to find a structured exercise program. A child without exercise may have a greater tendency toward obesity in later life because his or her body has developed *more and larger fat cells*. If that same child were exercising on a regular basis, he would have *fewer and smaller fat cells* and much less difficulty with his diet and weight when he becomes an adult. It has been estimated that 80 percent of obese children will be obese adults! It appears we do our children no favor by allowing them to eat and not exercise. Do you think they will thank you for allowing them to become fat adults?

We should instill in our children a love of sports by teaching techniques and skills. Regular trips to parks or outdoor events that require fresh air and walking are also helpful. Little league sports can be very helpful if the child is encouraged to enjoy the activity rather than placing the emphasis on winning. Remember, the goal is exercising and establishing a way of life, not being a member of an undefeated team that gets a trophy, which is put on the shelf to collect dust.

If Mom or Dad takes one of the children jogging with him or her, a few things must be kept in mind. Parents usually take one step to the child's two; thus, in reality they are asking the child to run twice as fast! Would any adult like to run at a doubled pace? Also the lung capacity of a child is much smaller than that of an adult. Therefore, the child is forced to breathe faster and harder when jogging. Jogging will become too hard if the child is forced to breathe fast for a long period of time. *Slow down* and run at a pace that the child can carry on a conversation.

Jogging is a great way to spend time with young children. Consider it a "time with my child" and then jog your own pace after your son or daughter has finished.

## 11. *Can I smoke and still jog?*

It always amazes me to talk with joggers who were once smokers. Jogging appears to be very helpful in breaking the smoking habit. People usually start smoking for two reasons: 1) Because one or both parents smoke, or 2) because of peer pressure—to become part of the gang. None of us were born with the inherited tendency to need tobacco to satisfy us physically or mentally.

Studies show that 10 percent of the smoking population continue their habit because of its stimulating effect, 10 percent because of the enjoyment of handling a cigarette, and 15 percent because it relaxes them. (6, 19) These are the groups that find it easiest to give up smoking. Jogging certainly can help the people who fall into this category. However, with those for whom smoking is a reliever of tension (30 percent of all smokers), a psychological addiction (25 percent), or a habit (10 percent), it will be harder to break the habit.

If you decide that you are going to turn the smoking problem over to God and quit all at once, expect some physiological symptoms of withdrawal for 7 to 14 days. Common symptoms are headaches, muscle cramps, restless nights, and irritability. God will help us overcome the symptoms of withdrawal if we submit to Him and try not to do it on our own willpower.

Heavy smokers often say they don't quit smoking for fear of gaining weight. (Over 60 percent of smokers have tried to quit and have gained weight.) It has been estimated that you would have to gain *100 pounds* to equal the harmful effects of smoking over one pack of cigarettes per day. Jogging can relieve the anxiety of wanting to eat by curbing your appetite. Research shows that people who jog have less desire to eat after jogging than when they don't jog. Needless to say, if you have a desire for a cigarette and that desire is filled with exercise instead of food, you will lose weight rather than gain weight as you break the smoking habit.

God will deliver you from smoking, the same as He will from food, if you really get down to business with Him.

12. *What about physicians and the advice we get from them concerning recommended physical activity and diet?*

James F. Fixx, in his book, *The Complete Book of Running*, states:

Most physicians are in no better shape than the rest of us. In Southern California, fifty-eight doctors were given physical exams. Most were found to be in poor physical condition. One out of five smoked, two out of three were overweight; one in four had high blood pressure; one in five had an abnormal electrocardiogram while exercising; more than half had high serum lipid levels. (24)

Fixx also says in the same book,

The under-exercised, coronary-prone physician sees himself as the authority on health matters. He tends to reflect to others his own life-style and thinks he is giving good, sound advice. Because he views himself as an authority figure, he finds it difficult to accept ideas foreign to his own concepts, especially when they differ radically from what he believes to be sound, conservative practice. (24)

In other words, physicians advise us to do as they say, not as they do! Perhaps the physician's position should be defended from the standpoint of education. Most medical schools are too involved teaching symptoms of existing disease and consequently don't allocate time in the curriculum for preventive medicine or the study of exercise.

It has been estimated that less than 10 percent of the medical schools have more than 10 hours of classroom material concerning nutrition and maintaining health. Doctors know that the diabetic patient should avoid certain foods, but when questioned in depth, have difficulty in recommending a balanced diet. Many physicians don't know the protein, carbohydrate, or fat content of an egg, let alone its caloric value. Perhaps medical schools need to realize that, given proper physical activity and eating habits, human beings live 15 to 18 years longer.

13. *Should I jog if I am sick or have a fever?*

Elevation of body temperature with any illness means that your body's metabolism has increased at rest and is using more oxygen. If the resting body requirements are increased, it is obvious that the amount of exercise we are able to do is decreased. Jogging is a good example. We may be able to jog a great deal with a normal temperature, but if our body temperature is raised our circulatory system already is working harder. Using the pulse rate as a guide, a person with a fever will reach a higher pulse rate with less exercise than he would normally. A good rule to follow: Endurance exercises should be curtailed if an individual has a temperature of 100°F or more.

Athletes can continue to do mild exercise as long as they do not overextend themselves.

### 14. *Is it OK to exercise with a cold?*

There is *no* good evidence that exposure to cold weather either makes a present cold worse or starts a new cold. You can exercise as long as your fever, if any, is below 100°F. If your temperature is higher, it should be down to normal and remain normal for 24 hours before you exercise again.

I personally am guilty of running even when I have a cold or don't feel good. My reasoning is that if I jog only a few minutes, my pulse rate is increased to the point where my sinuses drain and I get relief. I have, however, on occasion, exercised too long and caused my resistance to become lowered, thus prolonging my cold. Use logic. Don't overdo, but think *about doing*.

### 15. *Should a woman exercise during her menstrual cycle?*

Most women occasionally experience bothersome symptoms related to their menstrual cycle. These symptoms may include cramps, depression, irritability, backache, nausea, weakness, a feeling of "heavy legs," or a feeling of being bloated due to water retention. Physicians suggest that women not exercise strenuously during the first two days of their menstrual period. A heavy flow may make exercise impractical, or severe cramping may make it uncomfortable. Most physicians agree, however, that reasonable exercise during menstruation is acceptable and actually helpful in relieving cramps. Exercise may also relieve irritability and other emotional symptoms associated with the menstrual cycle.

### 16. *How can I guard against shin splints?*

Shin splints are an inflammation in the muscles and tendons that cover the shinbone in the front of the lower leg. Shin splints are caused by insufficient warm-up stretching exercises, by improper footwear, or by running too high on your toes.

To strengthen your shin muscles, sit on the edge of a table and hang a five-pound weight (a paint can with rocks or sand works nicely) on the lower part of the foot just above the toes. Raise your toes slowly, keep them up for a few seconds, and then lower your foot. Repeat the exercise until the shin muscles feel tired. Do not move your lower leg during this exercise, only your foot in an up-and-down motion.

### 17. *What do I do about "side stitch"?*

A side stitch (cramp) occurs while you are running hard enough to require deep breathing for a long time. It usually will disappear if you run more slowly. It is interesting to note that well-conditioned athletes seldom get a side stitch. Thus, the better shape you are in, the less chance of a side stitch.

However, if you do get a side stitch, remember that the pain can do no harm to your body or your ability to breathe. Just breathe deeply *using your stomach muscles* and run more slowly. Sometimes, if you hold your breath and apply a pressure in your lungs for a period of two to three seconds, this speeds up getting rid of the pain.

Dr. George Sheehan says the stitch is due to diaphragm spasm. In his words, "Man's perfectly designed ventilatory system is being mishandled by its owner." (59)

The most obvious maltreatment is the sudden prolonged use of the diaphragm in a sedentary individual. The diaphragm is accustomed to moving 1.5 centimeters 18 times per minute while we are at rest. Exercise can cause an increase up to 7 centimeters at a rate of 45 breaths per minute. Such demand on an unconditioned muscle explains why this occurs so often in beginning runners and middle-aged joggers.

There is an exercise that you can use at home to help prevent side stitch. Lie on the floor with a book on your stomach. Breathe with your stomach so that the book rises as you breathe inward. It is good to make a habit of breathing out against a slight resistance.

18. *What about tendonitis?*

There are some general principles which I feel apply to most cases of tendonitis of the foot, ankle, or knee. Most problems of tendonitis begin with an improper foot strike, improper footwear (shoes and/or socks), or attempts to jog too fast a pace for the current level of physical conditioning.

Jog by striking the heel first, then roll through the arch and push off with the toes. Flat-footed running can cause pain to knee joints. If the problem persists, I recommend jogging on a surface other than a paved road. Try jogging on slightly firm grass or the tree bark of park hiking paths where the terrain is fairly level.

Following each period of jogging, immerse the affected area in an ice bath or place an ice bag on it for approximately 10, preferably 20 minutes. In severe cases repeat the ice treatment three to four times a day. One or two five-grain aspirin can also be taken one to three times a day to help dull the aching.

If the pain persists after trying the above treatments, I recommend resting from jogging for a few days. Sometimes rest is just what is needed to help us get over a hump in retraining fatty muscles.

A major recommendation is to find a sports-oriented podiatrist and have him analyze your foot strike and running stride. On the basis of this analysis he will be able to provide you with the foot stabilization that is necessary.

### 19. *Do sit-ups help take off rolls around our waist?*

Sit-ups alone will not decrease the fat roll around our middle. That roll is subcutaneous fat that has permeated our entire body, not just the stomach muscles under the roll of fat. If we lose body fat in general, the waist roll will decrease proportionately. (53)

Spot reducers, such as pulley belts and rollers, are useless. Do we honestly think these belts or wooden rollers can break up "midriff bulge"? It amazes me that the machines are manufactured and actually sold for a profit. They are of zero value in reducing body fat.

### 20. *How often must I exercise to stay fit?*

Covert Bailey states the following in his book, *Fit or Fat*:
- Fitness is lost if you exercise two or less days per week.
- Fitness is maintained if you exercise three days per week. This, of course, is after you are in good shape. If you are in poor shape and only exercise three days per week it will be very difficult for you to maintain fitness.
- Fitness is improved if you exercise four or more days per week. (9)

Dr. Ken Cooper says you must exercise four days per week to maintain healthy muscle tissue. I suggest six days per week, because this allows for the greatest possibility of improvement and still gives you one day of rest.

### 21. *Is lifting weights good for weight control?*

Weight training is a reliable and safe method of building and maintaining muscle mass. Muscle mass is important to your health and energy level. We should think of our muscle cells as the energy cells of the body. The muscle cells release energy from food we eat. Individuals with deteriorated muscle mass, such as the overweight, over-fat, or out of shape, have a low energy level. Lack of muscle mass makes it easier to gain fat, despite calorie restriction below recommended levels for proper nutrition.

Use a weight training program that meets your individual goal. A weight training program can develop either bulky muscles or smaller, firm muscles. Most adults, however, are not interested in building bulky muscles. Bulk, or a large mass of muscle tissue, is developed by lifting heavy weights with few repetitions. Mr. America contestants usually work out two to three hours per day with weights. Building strong, firm muscle tissue is accomplished by lifting lighter weights with a number of repetitions. Lifting weights does not require much time per week to develop and maintain the muscle firmness you desire. I personally lift enough weight to do 7–10 repetitions of each exercise. If I can do more than 10 repetitions easily, I increase the weight.

Healthy, well-developed muscle mass helps maintain good posture as well as a pleasing appearance. Loss of muscle mass is associated with aging or the beer belly syndrome, while good musculature is associated with a youthful, healthy appearance.

As muscle mass decreases less energy is used, even at rest. Age should have nothing to do with muscle mass. A pound of lean muscle in use by a 16-year-old competing athlete requires the same number of calories as a pound of lean muscle of a 60-year-old man no longer as active in sports. However, most adults do not maintain lean muscle mass as they get older. Many older people let their body muscles decrease in size from lack of activity or regular exercise. As their muscles decrease in size their body weight becomes fat. Fat tissue does not use nearly as many calories as muscle tissue when the body is at rest or during normal everyday functions. Most people become fat as they grow older not because of what they eat or because of lack of activity, but because they use less calories at rest than they used to use when they had more muscle mass. Ancel Keys showed that a decrease in the use of *calories at rest*, not age, is directly related to loss of muscle mass. (44)

Anyone who has done much weight training soon learns that when he is tired he cannot lift as much weight as when he is fresh. One of the first signs of muscle fatigue is loss of strength. Don't attempt to jog a long time and then, feeling tired, attempt to lift weights. I suggest you select the two days per week that you jog the least amount of time for your weight training days. Lifting lighter weights with 7–10 repetitions should allow you sufficient strength both to jog and exercise your muscle mass. If you are interested in building bulky muscles, perhaps you should not jog the same day that you lift weights, since the buildup of lactic acid from running will interfere with a heavy weight-training program.

Most weight training exercises that emphasize strength rather than bulk of muscle tissue require very little time to accomplish. Most people do muscle mass exercises in 15–20 minutes or less. Remember, jogging helps get your muscle mass into shape by reducing the fat content of the muscle. Lifting weights builds muscle mass by increasing the size of the individual muscle cells.

Weight training does very little for your cardiopulmonary

system. Jogging is still the best exercise for obtaining cardiopulmonary health and is also the fastest way to get back into shape. However, proper weight training can more quickly allow you to get your muscle mass into shape. Weight training will speed up weight loss by increasing muscle mass, which burns more calories at rest.

## 22. *What is interval training?*

Interval training is used by runners to help improve their speed for racing purposes. Dr. Woldemar Gerschler and Dr. Herbert Reiner of Germany, who pioneered the interval system in the 1930s, argue that runners gain endurance by repeatedly running short distances at high speed, and taking short breaks with incomplete recovery. (25)

Dr. Edward Fox and Dr. Donald Mathews, who are in charge of the Exercise Physiology Research Laboratory at Ohio State University, wrote a book entitled *Interval Training*. Fox and Mathews feel that interval training can be done basically two different ways to help the athlete. One way is to run a specific distance in a period of time with a specific period of rest before another training time. (25)

Listed below is an example used in their book:

Set 1           6 × 220 at 0:33 (1:39)
Where:          6 = number of repetitions
              220 = training distance in yards
             0:33 = training time in minutes and seconds
            (1:39) = time of rest interval in minutes and seconds

The training athlete runs 220 yards in 33 seconds and then walks or jogs gently for 1 minute 39 seconds. (This is a 1 to 3 ratio of running to resting.) The athlete does this six times to equal one set of interval training.

The second form of interval training is based on the *heart rate response* during the work interval. For a young man or woman athlete less than 20 years of age, a heart rate of 190 beats per minute during the work interval is considered a sufficient work rate. Then, the heart is allowed to return to 125-150 beats per minute before running another work interval.

Fox and Mathews feel that a 40-year-old man or woman who is in *good* physical condition can run a work interval period of exercise to get the heart rate up to 160 beats per minute. They recommend that the pulse rate return to 105-120 beats per minute before starting a new work interval.

Intervals help the runner to increase the body's ability to run with oxygen debt and to learn to run hard in a state of fatigue. The usual interval distances are 100, 220, and 440 yards.

I feel that interval training is best suited for the athlete who is in running competition. Most adults who have gotten out of shape can hurt themselves by using interval training methods. Adults who have little body fat, a healthy lean body mass, and who have been jogging for a long time can alter their exercise programs with interval training. To someone who is just starting to jog, *I suggest you wait at least a year before attempting interval training methods.*

### 23. *What is a stress electrocardiogram?*

Suppose you were going to buy a used tractor to plow the ground for a garden. Would you go to look at the tractor, make sure the motor would start, and then pay for the tractor? Or would you want to see the tractor and plow demonstrated to make sure it could till the soil? Just as the tractor must plow under stress, your heart should be tested under stress to make sure it can function properly and without risk during exercise.

Have you ever heard of a patient getting a complete

physical examination, his physician informing him he is in good health, and before the patient can put his key in the ignition of his car he has a heart attack and dies? All of the tests, including a resting EKG, showed his heart to be in good shape. Sound familiar? A clean bill of health after a physical without a stress or exercise EKG is *not* a clean bill of health. We need to "plow the field" to make sure the heart has the capability to perform under stress.

A stress EKG should be done on a motorized treadmill where the amount of exercise a person performs can be precisely controlled, along with monitoring the individual's heartbeat and blood pressure during the exercise period. At the Dallas Cooper Clinic Dr. Ken Cooper uses a treadmill speed of 3.3 miles per hour and then raises the incline one percent per minute during the exercise period. After 25 minutes, the incline stays the same (25 percent) and the speed is increased 0.2 mph per minute. (19) As the patient works harder, heartbeat and blood pressure are carefully monitored. The exercise EKG should be continued to the point where the maximal heart rate (MHR) for the individual patient can be determined. The patient must be pushed to capacity in order to make the test valid.

There is a small chance that an individual being tested during a stress EKG could have a heart attack. The people conducting the test should be qualified in reading EKG's and be able to recognize a problem as it occurs. But it is better to have a heart problem arise under testing conditions with a cardiologist present than when driving a car on a busy freeway.

The American Heart Association has recently taken a stand that a submaximal heart stress test (80 percent MHR) is sufficient in evaluating the heart's performance. (3) Yet, Dr. Cooper, who has tested 26,000 patients, feels only a maximal stress test is valid. His statistics show that 12 percent of patients tested did not show heart disease until the patient had reached 90 percent of his MHR. Dr. Cooper, to my knowledge, has tested the hearts of more patients than anyone else to date. I feel the American Heart Association will soon realize that maximal heart testing is the best test to show the condition of the heart.

### 24. *How fast can my heart beat?*

How high should your heartbeat be elevated in order to give your heart's performance an adequate stress test? Depending on your age and condition, there is a limit to how fast your heart will go, no matter how long or hard you exercise. We call this *maximum heart rate.* The maximum heart rate *decreases with age,* as you can see by Tables 7 and 8 which are figures taken from the book, *The Complete Book of Running* by Jim Fixx. (24)

These figures are an *average* of many people in specific age categories. Of course, the only way to know your own maximum heart rate is to have a stress test yourself. Also

Table 7. Optimum Heartbeat Rate During Exercise: Women

| | Heartbeats Per Minute | | |
|---|---|---|---|
| *Age* | *Minimum with Exercise* | *Maximum with Exercise** | *Optimum or 80% MHR* |
| 25 | 130 | 185 | 148 |
| 30 | 126 | 180 | 144 |
| 35 | 123 | 175 | 140 |
| 40 | 119 | 170 | 136 |
| 45 | 116 | 165 | 132 |
| 50 | 112 | 160 | 128 |
| 55 | 109 | 155 | 124 |
| 60 | 105 | 150 | 120 |
| 65 | 102 | 145 | 116 |

*Dr. Ken Cooper's book, *The Aerobic Way,* gives slightly higher readings for maximal heart rate.

Table 8. Optimum Heartbeat Rate During Exercise: Men

| Age | Heartbeats Per Minute | | |
|---|---|---|---|
| | Minimum with Exercise | Maximum with Exercise* | Optimum or 80% MHR |
| 25 | 137 | 195 | 156 |
| 30 | 133 | 190 | 152 |
| 35 | 130 | 185 | 148 |
| 40 | 126 | 180 | 144 |
| 45 | 123 | 175 | 140 |
| 50 | 119 | 170 | 136 |
| 55 | 116 | 165 | 132 |
| 60 | 112 | 160 | 128 |
| 65 | 109 | 155 | 124 |

*Dr. Ken Cooper's book, *The Aerobic Way*, gives slightly higher readings for maximal heart rate.

keep in mind that the above figures are based on a resting heart rate of 72 for males and 80 for females. Since my resting heart rate is in the mid-40s and my age is 43, I cannot accurately use the above table. After stress testing my maximum heart rate was recorded at 170.

There is a formula that can be used to approximate your maximum heart rate. Needless to say, it is not totally accurate but it is helpful until you have a stress test completed. I first saw this formula in Covert Bailey's book, *Fit or Fat*. (9)

(Maximum–Resting) 65% + Resting =

Training Heart Rate (80% MHR)

Example: (180–62 = 118) × .65 = 76.7 + 62 = 138

Let's work through an example: Your average resting heart rate is 62 and you are 40 years old. Maximum for a fair conditioned 40-year-old male is 180. 180 minus 62 equals 118. 65% of 118 equals 76.7. 76.7 plus 62 equals 138. Your exercise rate, which is 80 percent of your maximum heart rate, should be 138-140. So when jogging, stop periodically and take your pulse. If it is above 140, slow your pace.

The Masters Double Step Test is *not* a stress test of your heart. This test has the patient step up and down a small two-step ladder. Then the patient lies down immediately and an electrocardiogram is recorded at different time intervals. The difficulty with this type of test is that it does not show an exercise EKG at all—only a recovery EKG after moderate exercise.

A complete cardiac examination consists of taking a thorough medical history, blood tests, listening to heart sounds through the chest, determining blood pressure, and monitoring your heart during rest and exercise with an electrocardiograph.

25. *What factors may rule out exercise?*

- Recent surgery
- Infectious diseases
- Kidney disease
- Fractures
- EKG abnormalities
- Extremely high blood pressure

If you have any doubts at all about your exercise program, be sure to call your physician—even if he smokes!

# CHAPTER 10

## Eating Right

Now we come to the place where I want to whet your appetite—not to *eat* more, but to *learn* more about the food you eat. I want to raise your level of consciousness concerning food: its value for energy; its potential for harm; and its potential for good. From this introductory material, may you be motivated to *read more* on your own and *gain a knowledge about food.*

### America's Favorite Pastime

Eliminating or preventing obesity is a major preoccupation in today's Western society. The reason is clear: Almost everyone enjoys eating. Many people entertain by having parties where food and drink are in abundance, while others celebrate by eating out at their favorite restaurant. Eating is a definite part of the social and business tradition of our American culture.

A person eats to achieve a certain satisfying sense of having filled his stomach. If it were not for the adverse effect of obesity on appearance and health, many people would probably eat even far more than they do.

The basis for a successful program of getting unwanted body fat off and keeping it off is a combination of exercise and restriction of food intake, as was shown by the Zuti and Golding study in Chapter 5. (69) It is eating foods that still satisfy your desire for food while not overloading the body with calories. In short, it is not willpower most people need, but *knowledge* of how to select natural foods and then prepare these foods properly. God can change our desire for food, but it is our responsibility to learn about food and its nutritional value. Again, the goal here is to highlight for you the whole realm of nutrition and encourage you to avail yourself of the many good books written on the subject. (A suggested reading list can be found at the end of this book.)

## How Do We Digest Food?

Digestion is one of the most fundamental functions of your body. Without it you would be unable to obtain any of the energy from the foods you eat. It is the process that converts all the food you eat to energy: good food, junk food, or anything you place in your mouth and swallow.

A good way to think of your entire digestive system, from the point where food enters the mouth until the unabsorbed residue leaves, is that it is a long hollow tube lined by specialized skin—let's call it your "internal skin." The specialized lining of the digestive tract is a barrier to the external environment, just as your outer skin is a barrier to cold weather. You can swallow a glass marble and it will pass through the entire digestive tube and never enter your body because it cannot be digested. You can swallow food, but unless it is broken down it will not enter your body and thus will not be used as energy for body functions.

## Start of Digestive Process

The digestive process begins even before you take the first bite of food from your plate. Just thinking about food, seeing food, or smelling food can start the process. If you have ever watched a dog drooling while looking at a juicy piece of meat or steak bone, you have observed the beginning of the digestive process. Not only does the saliva start to run, but if you could see the stomach you would see it start to churn and see an increase in the flow of digestive juices.

The mechanical breakdown of solid foods begins with the

chewing action. As you chew your food, it is lubricated with saliva to make it easier to swallow. If you eat a slice of bread or a baked potato, enzymes in the saliva (ptyalin or amylase) start breaking it down into small units. There isn't time for much digestion to take place in the mouth, but the initial breakdown continues as you swallow your food.

The solid foods you eat are literally milked down the esophagus (because of the lubricant effect of the saliva) to the stomach by the rhythmic squeezing actions of your esophagus. It doesn't take very long for the food to arrive at the inlet to your stomach. The stomach door then opens to accept the wetted solid food chunks. By contrast, fluid, especially water, passes down the esophagus as fast as you can swallow it. (Kind of like pouring water down a tube.) There is nothing to stop the water and it quickly passes the sphincter (valve) of the stomach and enters the small intestine. There are no important digestive actions in the esophagus.

## Function of the Stomach

The stomach is primarily a storage pouch or food reservoir. Very little food is absorbed from the stomach into your system. Water passes almost immediately around any solid bolus (ball of food) you may have in your stomach and into the first part of the small intestine, the duodenum. Absorption in the small intestine is about 10 times more rapid than in the stomach. About 95 percent of the water that enters the stomach is completely absorbed into your bloodstream in less than 10 minutes.

It is important to note that your stomach will not allow solid food to pass into the small intestine. The solids are partially digested, churned, and mixed with liquid secretions from the stomach, forming a liquid or semi-solid slush. As the outer shell of the bolus is broken down, the liquid material is squirted out of the stomach into the duodenum. Therefore, a liquid meal passes quickly, and a meal with bulk stays in the stomach for as long as it takes to liquify.

Your stomach processes carbohydrates more quickly than proteins or fats. The scale runs from refined sugar, such as sweetened soft drinks, that move through the stomach quickly, to a raw apple, which is slowly converted to slush and emptied from the stomach. This is important to you because the bulky carbohydrates prevent overloading of your blood with rapidly absorbed glucose. The blood glucose level hardly rises if you eat a raw apple, because of the reservoir effect of your stomach and the slow release of the apple into your intestine. Bulk, whether it comes from raw vegetables, fruit, or cereal fiber, is important in helping to control your blood sugar level. (56) In the person who eats simple starch as found in enriched breads and concentrated sweets, or drinks sweet liquids, glucose is absorbed rapidly and the blood sugar rises quickly to a high level.

Proteins are processed less rapidly than carbohydrates. If you ingest protein as a gelatin-mix drink it passes fairly quickly through the digestive system, but if it is a solid meat it must be "slushed" before it can leave the stomach for absorption. Fat markedly slows stomach emptying. A fatty meal has been demonstrated to remain in a dog's stomach as long as 24 hours after it has been ingested. (34) As the fat leaves your stomach and enters the small intestine, it causes a hormone (enterogastrone) to be released that inhibits the stomach contractions and slows its emptying. Clearly, if you are in need of instant energy, you should not eat *any* fat.

## Where the Action Is!

The small intestine is really where the action is. The food slush from your stomach is acid, but when it enters the small intestine it is exposed to copious amounts of alkaline digestive juices. A major portion of these juices come from the wall of your small intestine.

All food slush that enters the small intestine must be broken down into the simplest form for absorption through the wall of the small intestine. That wall is over two millimeters thick, so it is not a simple membrane. Food particles do not simply diffuse across the intestinal wall but must be transported across the wall in a series of complex chemical steps.

Carbohydrates are broken down to double sugars (maltose, lactose, sucrose) by the enzymes from the saliva and pancreas and then must be broken down to the three single sugars (glucose, fructose, and galactose) before they can be transported across the intestinal wall. It makes no difference whether the double sugar comes from a raw apple or refined sugar, the end result is the same. The enzymes that accomplish this final breakdown are from the wall of the intestine itself. The final breakdown results in the three single sugars actually entering your bloodstream. A similar thing happens to protein. The small combinations of amino acids are finally broken down into their basic amino acids, which are absorbed through the intestinal wall.

You will find it interesting to know that your digestive system's lining acts like your external skin and sheds regularly. Your small intestine has a complete *new lining every three days*. To accomplish this shedding act your small intestine sheds about a half-pound (250 grams) of cells each day. (34) These are broken down in your small intestine, digested into amino acids, and transported through the intestinal wall with the amino acids from your food. The amino acids in these cells are no different from the amino acids in your food and are just as useful. Your body is an excellent example of a recycling machine.

Once food residue has passed through the small intestine into the colon (large intestine), *digestion stops*. The main function of the colon is to reabsorb any fluid that may need to be absorbed, thus preserving the body's water balance. Salt and water are both affected by this action. (Diarrhea results in a loss of water and salts, causing a body imbalance.)

## Calories Do Count!

Preparing good food that is not fattening depends on knowing which foods contain the most calories. Make no mistake about it—*calories do count.* It doesn't make any difference whether a calorie is in a protein food, a fat food, or a carbohydrate food. *A calorie is a calorie* and it is a unit of energy. Remember that energy can neither be created nor destroyed. If you swallow and absorb a calorie your body must process it. You will use it for energy or store it as fat.

Food is made up of water, undigestible bulk, calories, minerals, and vitamins. Water content and undigestible bulk are major factors in determining how many calories are in any food. A good example is raw round steak. After all the visible fat is removed, the remaining meat is over 70 percent water. That is why a whole pound of lean round steak contains only about 600 calories.

Fish is about 80 percent water and is a low calorie food. Fresh fruits and vegetables contain lots of water. Many vegetables, particularly those used for salads, contain lots of water and undigestible bulk. That is why raw lettuce is such a low calorie food. Whole milk is 87 percent water. Most of the foods you use are calories diluted with water and undigestible bulk, whether they be solid (such as meat) or liquid (such as milk or fruit juice).

*The high calorie foods are those which contain little water or undigestible bulk.* Sugar is a good example. Less than one percent of its weight is water. One hundred grams (three and one-half ounces) of sugar contains 385 calories. The same weight of raw, lean round steak contains only 135 calories. Sugar contains almost three times as many calories.

Foods are divided into *carbohydrates, fats,* and *proteins. Fat* is the highest calorie food. Lard is a good example as it contains no water. One hundred grams of lard contain 902 calories. *A gram of fat contains nine calories while a gram of protein or carbohydrate contains about four calories.* Calories are important, but the body also needs the water and undigestible bulk found in food items. The various cooking oils contain no water; consequently 100 grams contain 884 calories, just slightly less than lard. It follows that a low-fat diet is usually a low-calorie diet. However, if we eat 100 calories more than our body needs it will be *stored as FAT*, no matter if it is fat, carbohydrate, or protein. Let's look at some specifics.

## Calories in Beef, Poultry, Fish

You can eat a lot of *meat* and not consume a lot of calories. Which meat you select and how it is prepared makes a lot of difference. Remove all the visible fat from the steak before cooking. If you do this you can eat 100 grams raw weight of the lean beef and consume only 130 to 150 calories, even if you choose flank steak, porterhouse steak, T-bone steak, club steak, sirloin steak, or round steak. If you choose a steak and eat it fat and all, the same weight of the edible portion provides 390 calories, over twice the calorie consumption. Meat with fat marbling is 30-60 percent fat. So remove all fat before eating meat.

*Poultry* is a great source of protein with limited calories. Chicken light meat without the skin contains the least calories (only 101 calories in 100 grams). If the skin is left on, the same amount contains 120 calories. Dark meat with skin contains 132 calories. Breast of chicken or young turkey is an excellent choice for good protein while limiting calories.

Roasting, broiling, or even boiling chicken results in fewer calories than frying it. Any frying process for beef, chicken, or fish adds fat and calories. Any breading, crumbing, or dredging merely provides a means of adding fat and un-needed calories to the basic dish. If you must fry, use pan broiling, which means frying on an elevated surface in a pan so that the fat drains away, keeping the meat from being soaked in grease.

*Fish*, as a group, tends to be low in calories, but what fish you choose makes a difference. Cod, flounder, and sole contain only 79 calories in 100 grams, while the same amount of salmon contains 217 calories. Rainbow trout contains 195 calories. The fish that contain the most calories have more fat in the meat. By avoiding salmon, lake trout, and sardines, you can eat a great deal of fish, if it is properly prepared, and not eat a lot of calories. To avoid extra calories, do not cook the fish in any form of batter. Broiling is the best choice. Don't eat it with ordinary tartar sauce, as this only adds calories. Add spices according to your taste—not butter or oil. Lemon adds a nice flavor to most fish.

### Low Calorie Fruit and Vegetable Group

*Vegetables* are low calorie foods. A 100-gram serving of cooked navy beans contains 118 calories. A similar weight of raw mature bean seeds contains 340 calories. The difference is in the water content. As the beans are cooked they swell with water and the 100-gram serving of cooked beans is nearly 70 percent water by weight. A baked or boiled potato with the skin removed contains only about 100 calories in 100 grams, but if milk and butter are added to make mashed potatoes, 100 grams contains 185 calories. It is not the potato but what is added to it that makes it high in calories.

A 100-gram serving of cooked green peas contains only 82 calories, but if you add a teaspoon of butter (which is not very much) you are adding 100 calories of fat and converting it into a high fat food. This is the usual story with vegetables. It is what you add that counts in terms of calories. It is better to avoid the fats and learn to use spices and low calorie sauces for flavor.

Most *fruits* are low in calories. Again, it is what you add to

the fruit that adds the calories. Learn to eat *raw fruit* and
you won't consume so many calories. Learn the caloric
content of fruit and you will discover you can eat a lot of pears
and apples without consuming a large amount of calories.

## Carbohydrates

There are two types of carbohydrates in our daily food
intake. One type is *simple*, the other *complex*. All carbohydrates, after being digested by the intestinal acids, become
the simple type of carbohydrate called glucose. The simple
carbohydrate breaks down very fast into glucose, whereas
the complex type takes much longer. As a matter of fact
some of the more complex carbohydrates, like cellulose,
hemicellulose, and lignin, are only partially digested and
serve as roughage material to help move food through the
intestinal tract.

*Simple carbohydrates* like table sugar (sucrose), lactose in
milk, and maltose become blood glucose very quickly. *Complex carbohydrates*, found in fruits, vegetables, and grains,
take a longer period of time to break down into blood glucose.
Most grains are good examples of slow- to almost nondigestible complex carbohydrates. The outer covering of
wheat, rye, oats, barley, or rice is mostly nondigestible by
our intestinal tract and acts as roughage. The most popular
item today is bran, which is nothing more than the outer
covering of wheat kernels. The inner part of the grain kernel
is a slow-digesting carbohydrate.

It is best if our carbohydrate daily allowance is from whole
grain breads and cereals, fruits, and vegetables, adding as
little fats and sweeteners as possible.

In general terms, strive for approximately 70 percent of
your caloric intake to come from the area of *complex* carbohydrates. This includes whole grain breads, whole grain
cereals, fruits, and vegetables. Only 25 percent of your total
calorie intake need come from the area of protein products,

such as fortified skim milk, lean meat, poultry, and seafood. It becomes obvious that fruits, such as pears, apples, bananas, plums, and oranges—and vegetables, such as corn, beans, carrots, celery, and lettuce, must be eaten in two of our three daily meals.

You owe it to yourself to learn more about the effect of simple and complex carbohydrates on your system. Why not try eating nothing but fruit for breakfast or lunch and notice how "good" you feel for three to four hours following your complex carbohydrate meal.

Table 9 reveals what various foods have to offer.

Table 9. Calories, Protein, Carbohydrates, and Fat in Foods*
(Per 100 Grams Edible Portion)

|  | Calories | Protein (grams) | Carbo-hydrates (grams) | Fat (grams) |
|---|---|---|---|---|
| Almonds, dried | 598 | 18.6 | 19.5 | 54.2 |
| Apples, raw, not pared | 58 | .2 | 14.5 | .6 |
| Applesauce, canned, unsweetened | 41 | .2 | 10.8 | .2 |
| Asparagus, fresh, cooked | 20 | 2.2 | 3.6 | .2 |
| Avocados, raw | 167 | 2.1 | 6.3 | 16.4 |
| Bamboo shoots, raw | 27 | 2.6 | 5.2 | .3 |
| Bananas | 85 | 1.1 | 22.2 | .2 |
| Beans, snap, fresh, cooked in water | 25 | 1.6 | 15.4 | .2 |
| T-bone steak, broiled | 473 | 19.5 | 0 | 43.2 |
| Ground beef, lean, cooked | 219 | 27.4 | 0 | 11.3 |
| Beets, fresh, cooked | 32 | 1.1 | 7.2 | .1 |
| Bread | | | | |
| White, enriched, with 2% nonfat dry milk | 269 | 8.7 | 50.4 | 8.7 |
| Rye | 243 | 9.1 | 52.1 | 1.1 |

|  | Calories | Protein (grams) | Carbo-hydrates (grams) | Fat (grams) |
|---|---|---|---|---|
| Whole-wheat, 2% nonfat dry milk | 243 | 10.5 | 47.7 | 3.0 |
| Cheese |  |  |  |  |
| Cheddar | 398 | 25.0 | 2.1 | 32.2 |
| Cottage, creamed | 106 | 13.6 | 2.9 | 4.2 |
| Swiss | 370 | 27.5 | 1.7 | 28.0 |
| Chicken |  |  |  |  |
| Light meat, cooked, without skin | 166 | 31.6 | 0 | 3.4 |
| Dark meat, cooked, without skin | 176 | 28.0 | 0 | 6.3 |
| Eggs, hard cooked | 163 | 12.9 | .9 | 11.5 |
| Lettuce, iceberg | 13 | .9 | 2.9 | .1 |
| Orange juice, raw | 45 | .7 | 10.4 | .2 |
| Perch, raw | 118 | 19.3 | 0 | 4.0 |
| Tomatoes, ripe, raw | 22 | 1.1 | 4.7 | .2 |
| Tuna, canned in water | 127 | 28.0 | 0 | .8 |
| Yoghurt, made from partially skimmed milk | 50 | 3.4 | 5.2 | 1.7 |

*Bernice K. Watt and Annabell L. Merrill, "Composition of Foods," *Agriculture Handbook No. 8* (Washington, D.C.: U.S. Government Printing Office).

## Success in Dieting Equals Knowledge of Food

All of the four basic food groups (breads and cereals, vegetables and fruits, meats, and dairy products) can be obtained as low calorie food items. If you prepare these low calorie items properly without adding fats or sugar, you can have a wide variety of foods and eat a large amount without consuming too many calories. Diet success is then achieved by what you do in the kitchen rather than by what you refuse at the table.

# Fat

Dietary fats are important for their palatability value, as a source of concentrated energy, as a carrier of the fat-soluble vitamins, and as a source of essential fatty acids. Of all the fatty acids, only one (linoleic acid) cannot be synthesized by our body and must be derived from food. The richest sources of lineoleic acid are vegetable oils; safflower has the most, followed by sunflower, corn, cottonseed, soybean, sesame, and peanut oil.

## *Three Types of Fat to be Aware Of*

1. *Saturated.* Hard at room temperature; primarily from animal sources—lard, butterfat, and the yellowish-white fat of muscle meats. Saturated fat from coconut oil and palm oil may also be found in imitation dairy products.

2. *Unsaturated or polyunsaturated.* Liquid at room temperature; found primarily in vegetable and seed oils. Grains, vegetables, and fruits generally contain more polyunsaturated fats than saturated fats.

3. *Hydrogenated.* Polyunsaturated fats that have been changed to solids or semisolids by the addition of hydrogen. This process essentially converts polyunsaturates to saturated fats. Hydrogenated fats are found in various processed foods, including shortening, margarine, some peanut butter, chip-type snack foods, and some candies.

No RDA (recommended daily allowance) has been set for fat, but many nutritionists believe we should derive no more than 35 percent of our total daily calories from fats. (I feel this is too high; 10 percent will supply us with enough of the essential fatty acids.) Americans not only exceed the 35 percent limit, but they also eat far more saturated animal fat than is healthy for them. Most health authorities are now advising Americans to sharply reduce the amount of fat in their diets, particularly saturated and hydrogenated fats.

## Sugar

Brothers and sisters, we have got "trouble in River City" in an area many of us are overlooking. The trouble is a white, crystalline substance that affects most everyone. This substance is not heroin, speed, or LSD; it is sugar.

Many Christians who avoid cigarettes or alcohol because they are harmful stuff themselves and their families with sugar, and all the while see nothing wrong with something as American as apple pie, or brownies, or . . . (insert your favorite dessert). But sugar, like hard drugs, provides the body with a lift; the "quick energy food" is how it is billed. What it also does, after the lift, is bring on a slump, which results in the need and desire for more and more sugar, another "fix"—a vicious cycle. The fact is that the average American now consumes around 140 pounds of refined sugar a year, up from seven pounds per person in 1900.

"Is it really so bad?" you may be asking. Dr. John Yudkin, in his book, *Sweet and Dangerous,* says:

Right at the outset I can make two key statements that no one can refute: first, there is no physiological requirement for sugar. All human nutritional needs can be met in full without having to take a single spoon of white or brown or raw sugar, on its own or in any food or drink. Secondly, if only a small fraction of what is already known about the effects of sugar were to be revealed in relation to any other material used as a food additive, the material would promptly be banned. (67)

By *sugar* we are referring to refined cane or beet sugar. Our Creator made the sugar cane with some 64 ingredients. We "improve" on His work by extracting out the B complex, enzymes, proteins, minerals, and vitamins, in the form of the black strap molasses. What is left is the refined substance we are all so familiar with, robbed of all the nourishment except calories. It is a dead food. Even worse, all forms of sugar raise the body's vitamin needs (vitamins are called on to "burn" the sugar, thereby depressing the vitamin supply) and cause blood chemistry disturbances. A word here about honey: If it is overdone it is just as bad as white sugar.

Carleton Fredericks, in his book, *Breast Cancer–A Nutritional Approach*, says,

How do you drift into a way of eating which sickens and kills animals, and crowds our hospitals and medical facilities? You begin by assuming that average is normal. What is more American than apple pie? There is nothing normal about a dessert which in one serving supplies 12 teaspoons of sugar, unless you take it a la mode, which brings the sugar total of 18 teaspoonfuls per portion. (27)

This is a good point to look at the amount of sugar in various foods. Some of the information in Table 10 may surprise you.

Table 10. Sugar in Beverages and Foods

| Item | Portion | Amount (Teaspoonfuls of granulated sugar) |
|---|---|---|
| *Beverages* | | |
| Cola drinks | 6 oz. | 3½ |
| Ginger ale | 6 oz. | 5 |
| Highball | 6 oz. | 2½ |
| Root beer | 10 oz. | 4½ |
| Seven-up | 6 oz. | 3¾ |
| Sweet cider | 1 cup | 6 |
| *Dairy products* | | |
| Ice cream cone | 1 | 3½ |
| Ice cream soda | 1 | 5 |
| Ice cream sundae | 1 | 7 |
| Malted milk shake | 10 oz. | 5 |
| *Desserts, miscellaneous* | | |
| Apple cobbler | ½ cup | 3 |
| Blueberry cobbler | ½ cup | 3 |

| Item | Portion | Amount (Teaspoonfuls of granulated sugar) |
|------|---------|-------------------------------------------|
| Custard | ½ cup | 2 |
| Fruit gelatin | ½ cup | 4½ |
| Apple pie | 1 slice (average) | 7 |
| Berry pie | 1 slice | 10 |
| Cherry pie | 1 slice | 10 |
| Cream pie | 1 slice | 4 |
| Lemon | 1 slice | 7 |
| Peach pie | 1 slice | 7 |
| Pumpkin pie | 1 slice | 5 |
| Rhubarb pie | 1 slice | 4 |
| Banana pudding | ½ cup | 2 |
| Bread pudding | ½ cup | 1½ |
| Chocolate pudding | ½ cup | 4 |
| Date pudding | ½ cup | 7 |
| Rice pudding | ½ cup | 5 |
| Tapioca pudding | ½ cup | 3 |
| Berry tart | 1 cup | 10 |
| Sherbet | ½ cup | 9 |

### Cakes and cookies

| Item | Portion | Amount |
|------|---------|--------|
| Angel food cake | 4 oz. piece | 7 |
| Applesauce cake | 4 oz. piece | 5½ |
| Cheese cake | 4 oz. piece | 2 |
| Chocolate cake (iced) | 4 oz. piece | 10 |
| Coffee cake | 4 oz. piece | 4½ |
| Cup-cake (iced) | 1 | 6 |
| Fruit cake | 4 oz. piece | 5 |
| Pound cake | 4 oz. piece | 5 |
| Strawberry shortcake | 1 serving | 4 |
| Brownies (unfrosted) | 1 (¾ oz.) | 3 |
| Macaroons | 1 | 6 |
| Oatmeal cookies | 1 | 2 |
| Sugar cookies | 1 | 1½ |
| Chocolate eclair | 1 | 7 |
| Cream puff | 1 | 2 |
| Donut (glazed) | 1 | 6 |

### Candies

| Item | Portion | Amount |
|------|---------|--------|
| Average choc. milk bar | 1 (1½ oz.) | 2½ |

| Item | Portion | Amount *(Teaspoonfuls of granulated sugar)* |
|------|---------|-----------------------------|
| Chewing gum | 1 stick | ½ |
| Chocolate mints | 1 | 2 |
| Fudge | 1 oz. square | 4½ |
| Gumdrop | 1 | 2 |
| Peanut brittle | 1 oz. | 3½ |
| *Canned fruits and juices* | | |
| Canned apricots | 4 halves and 1 T syrup | 3½ |
| Canned fruit juices (sweet) | ½ cup | 2 |
| Canned peaches | 2 halves and 1 T syrup | 3½ |
| Fruit salad | ½ cup | 3½ |
| *Jams and jellies* | | |
| Apple butter | 1 T | 1 |
| Jelly | 1 T | 4-6 |
| Strawberry jam | 1 T | 4 |

*Information in this table is from Gly-Oxide, distributed by Marion Laboratories, Inc., 10236 Bunker Ridge Road, Kansas City, Missouri 64137.

If you have managed to avoid most of the items you still may be consuming sugar of which you are not even aware. It is present in most processed foods, such as ketchup, mayonnaise, relish, canned soups and vegetables, boxed cereals, salad dressings, and sadly, baby foods. Start reading labels and see for yourself. It has been estimated that 92 percent of everything we buy at the supermarket contains sugar.

## What Sugar Does in Us

Dr. E. Cheraskin says he would like to see printed on all candy wrappers the following warning: "This product can be dangerous to your mental health." (16) He is referring, of course, to the effects of eating too much refined sugar, associated with hypoglycemia or low blood sugar.

If that seems confusing, let us review briefly what happens when we eat sugar. The pancreas is the organ which produces the hormone insulin, and insulin regulates the concentration of sugar in the bloodstream. When you eat a meal the level of the blood sugar rises temporarily. This stimulates the pancreas to produce insulin to regulate the amount of blood sugar, and the blood sugar level then drops to a normal level. However, in some individuals, if they have been overloading their bloodstream with enormous amounts of refined sugars, there comes a time when this mechanism goes haywire. The pancreas becomes supersensitive and produces too much insulin.

Perhaps you are familiar with a diabetic who has had an insulin reaction, when he or she inadvertently took too much insulin. The result is a fall of the blood sugar level to an abnormally low level. Dr. Cheraskin says, in *Psychodietetics:*

Hypoglycemia is the exact opposite of diabetes; yet it is often the forerunner of that disease. In diabetes, too little usable insulin circulates in the bloodstream; in hypoglycemia (also called hyperinsulinism), there is too much. An excess of this sugar regulating hormone, released by the pancreas in response to a rapidly rising blood sugar, drives the blood sugar levels below normal, triggering a craving for sweets along with a variety of physical or mental symptoms. (16)

What are some of the symptoms? Headaches, fatigue or exhaustion, trouble getting started without sugar or caffeine, irritability, sweating, dizziness, fast and/or noticeable heartbeat, confusion, trembling, and others. It has been estimated that as much as one-fifth of the U.S. population suffers from this disease. (1, 16, 67)

It is a vicious cycle. Excessive consumption of sweets

triggers the release of too much insulin, the blood sugar drops to a level lower than before, and the symptoms of low blood sugar arrive, sending the individual looking for something sweet to relieve the fatigue, shakiness, or whatever. And remember, as if this isn't bad enough, hypoglycemia is often the forerunner of diabetes, the lack of sufficient insulin to handle sugar. Could it be the pancreas has been exhausted by all the demands of the "sugaraholic"? Not the best stewardship of the temple of the Holy Spirit, is it?

Hypoglycemia is not the only problem associated with excessive sugar consumption. Dr. John Yudkin, in *Sweet and Dangerous*, states: "My research on coronary disease has convinced me beyond doubt that sugar plays a considerable part in this terrifying modern epidemic." (67)

Dental decay is a direct result of a bad effect of sugar. Food containing sugar sticks to the tooth. Bacteria reacts with the sticky sugar and forms an acid which dissolves the tooth enamel. Think of the money that could have been saved in dental treatment, not to mention the unnecessary pain that is a part of dental disease.

An article in the August 24, 1977, *Medical Tribune*, stated that research in several countries has shown that overeating of sugar causes not only an increase of blood fats, like triglycerides, but also of blood concentrations of uric acid, diminished glucose tolerance leading to diabetes and low blood sugar, and increased adhesiveness of certain blood cells suggestive of conditions leading to strokes.

The following, according to most researchers, are some of the disorders at least partially caused by overeating sugar: (1, 22, 56, 67)

| | |
|---|---|
| Diabetes | Coronary thrombosis |
| Hypoglycemia | Blood chemistry disturbances |
| Mental problems | Increased dental disease |
| Obesity | Malnutrition |

### Just a Spoonful of Sugar . . .

Something needs to be said here about our children and their early exposure to sugar. Rewards for good behavior are often cookies, candies, and cakes, and the child is conditioned at an early age to become a sugar addict. If you doubt the severity of the situation, watch the reaction of your children when you announce that you are going to start changing the family diet for the better and eliminate junk food and desserts. At first there will be much howling, and very little interest in fresh fruits. ("Train up a child in the way he should go, [and] even when he is old . . ." [Prov. 22:6].)

Dr. Yudkin says,

Man always wanted to eat sweet foods because he liked them. So long as the only sweet foods he could find were fruit, by satisfying his wants for sweetness he helped to satisfy his needs for vitamin C and other nutrients. But since he began to produce his own foods, and especially since he developed the technology of sugar refining and food manufacture, he has been able to produce and separate sweetness from all nutrients. What he wants is no longer necessarily what he needs. (67)

It is my conclusion that our heavenly Father intended us to satisfy our desire for sweets with fruits. Period. And fruits the way *He* made them, not sugared and cooked and baked into a pie. It is impossible to sit down and eat 20 apples at a sitting; yet how much apple pie and ice cream can some people eat?

What's the answer? Simple, really. Get back to the diet the all-wise Creator intended for us. Fresh fruits and occasionally dried fruits are sweet enough. We like to have our palates tickled, rather than to eat nutritiously. However, it is possible to gradually wean yourself and your family off sugar, decreasing or cutting in half what is called for in recipes.

Along that line, let me quote Carleton Fredericks again, "All this brings you face to face with a resigned acceptance of the fact that you must reduce sugar to the status of a condiment. You don't use salt and pepper by the pound; why do you then accept recipes which begin with 'Take 2 cups of sugar'?" (27) And I might add, why do you then bring these desserts to a church supper, realizing this is not the way our Lord wants us to eat?

I suggest reading more about this subject and invite your attention to the bibliography and reading list at the end of the book. Remember, in the realm of self-control, the hardest step is the first one: deciding to subdue the flesh. We tend to want to put that off until later. But praise God, when we mean business, His help is there.

### Organic, Natural—Are They Best For You?

Have you noticed the word *natural* as part of a brand name? Have you noticed a sign saying that food was grown *organically*? As the terms *natural* and *organic* are being used more often, we need to understand their meaning.

The word *natural* refers to the character of the ingredients (no preservatives or artificial additives) and the fact that the food product has undergone minimal processing. The word *organic* refers to the way food has been grown (without chemicals in the form of fertilizers or pesticides).

### Natural

Supermarket shelves are being stocked with so-called natural products, some containing no preservatives while others contain many chemical additives. Food labels which read *natural* or *natural ingredients* or *few additives* should be questioned and perused with caution.

The safety of food additives or chemical preservatives should be considered when buying food items. Chemicals, while they prevent or retard spoilage in some foods, are not easily broken down and removed as a waste product by our bodies. Chemicals have no food value or vitamins and are definitely harmful when ingested over a long period of time. If food labels are read carefully we can find many foods in supermarkets that have been processed without additives.

The word *natural* does not guarantee healthy food. The food industry is adding *natural* to almost every type of food label and making us pay a higher price as well. For example, you can buy a brand of "natural" potato chips or a "natural" candy bar. The potato chips contain a chemical preservative, and the candy bar is so concentrated with sugar that a preservative is not needed.

The "natural" bandwagon has reached beyond the supermarket shelves. You can use "natural" soap to wash your dishes or "natural" shampoo to wash your hair or feed your dog a "natural" dog food. All of these items use the word *natural* but are full of chemical additives. We must take time to read the labels of food and other items that are ingested by our bodies.

## Organic

The desire to eat foods that do not contain pesticide residues makes considerable sense. Insecticides, herbicides, and fungicides are chemicals which have been reported possibly to cause cancer, birth defects, or reproductive disorders. How much of these chemicals we safely can ingest is not definitely known.

The term *organic* implies a specific way that fruits or vegetables have been grown. The produce is not subjected to any pesticides, fertilizers, or chemicals. The soil has been treated with natural fertilizers, such as manure or compost.

Organic enthusiasts believe that growing crops without the use of chemicals results in products more healthful and nutritious, containing more vitamins and minerals. Organic produce usually are more expensive to purchase. There is not yet enough scientific evidence to show that the nutrient content of organically grown plants is better than the nonorganically grown produce. (18) Plants derive their nutrients from the soil. The plant is not able to discern if the nutrients came from a chemical fertilizer or manure.

If soil is deficient of a certain mineral, that mineral can be added with a chemical fertilizer or realized by decomposition of manure. Manure usually is not a well-balanced fertilizer. It is often high in phosphate and low in nitrogen, and it can contain bacteria, insects or worms, and even toxic chemicals that were added to the animal's diet.

Enthusiasts take their stand that organic produce contain no pesticide residues. Unfortunately, laboratory tests over the years have shown little difference in the level of pesticide residues between organic produce and those grown commercially. Tests have also shown that farmers wishing to convert land to organic growing find that chemicals already in the soil can be detected in the plants for several years.

Common logic tells us that we should eat food that is grown with the least amount of chemicals. However, it is almost impossible for us to determine chemical content by looking at fruits and vegetables we purchase. It is also questionable whether we should pay a higher price for organic produce. However, produce always should be washed thoroughly and wiped before it is eaten.

# CHAPTER 11

## Vitamins and Minerals

### Vitamins

While all foods contain some vitamins, no vitamins contain proteins, carbohydrates, or fats. Vitamins are organic substances that help regulate bodily functions. Acting as coenzymes, vitamins aid the metabolism of food nutrients.

About a dozen major vitamins have been identified, though more may yet be discovered. A deficiency in any one essential vitamin produces a corresponding deficiency disease, generally (though not always) reversible when the missing vitamin is supplied again. Though present in small amounts, vitamins are crucial to the body's digestive, reproductive, nervous, and muscle systems. Vitamins also affect tissue growth and antibody production.

Whether you derive adequate vitamins from your diet or not depends on environmental factors, your individual needs, the amount of food you eat, and the composition of your diet. Whole, unprocessed foods are the best source of all known and unknown vitamins. Junk foods fill you up with calories and very little vitamins and minerals.

### An Overview of Identified Vitamins

VITAMIN A is important to eye health and a healthy condition of skin and mucous membranes. Sources include whole milk; egg yolks; butter; margarine; and yellow, yellowish red, and green fruits and vegetables (carrots, sweet potatoes, kale, tomatoes, apricots, spinach, and dandelion greens). Little vitamin A is found in meats, vegetable oils, nuts, or grains. Vitamin A is a fat-soluble vitamin and is stored by the body.

VITAMIN C is probably the most controversial vitamin. Its most avid boosters believe vitamin C cures or alleviates everything from colds and tennis elbow to cancer. More conservative followers acknowledge only that the vitamin is essential, that it prevents scurvy, that its presence helps form and maintain the protein of connective tissues, and that it influences wound-healing and metabolic functions. Vitamin C is water-soluble, easily lost in cooking water or by oxidation after harvest. Sources include vegetables and fruits, especially citrus fruits, tomatoes, green peppers, leafy greens, broccoli, cabbage, kale, rose hips, melons, mangos, brussel sprouts, cauliflower, and potatoes. Animal-origin foods have little or no vitamin C.

I personally take 500-1000 milligrams per day of vitamin C because I feel it helps prevent colds. Vitamin C appears to have tremendous value in helping metabolize food, as well as preventing disease. Read about this vitamin. It really does help.

VITAMIN D is fat-soluble, stored by the body, and is crucial for the absorption and utilization of calcium and phosphorus. Adequate vitamin D is as important to pregnant women and the unborn child as it is to young children; growing bones and teeth need plenty of calcium and phosphorus. A deficiency will cause rickets (soft bones) in children, producing deformed bone structure. Vitamin D is called the "sunshine vitamin." Exposing the skin to sunlight causes a chemical reaction in the skin oils, creating vitamin D that is eventually absorbed into the system. Food sources include liver, butter, egg yolks, and milk. Fortified milk has 400 IU of synthetic vitamin D added per quart. (Pasteurization of milk destroys the natural vitamin D so it must be added to the milk.)

VITAMIN E's specific importance to human physiology is

not yet fully understood. Some authorities feel that vitamin E (alpha tocopherol) may be a cure for and prophylactic against heart disease. Others say it can improve sexual function or slow down the aging process. Vitamin E is known to be an antioxidant that acts to protect the body's store of vitamins A and C and unsaturated fatty acids. Sources include wheat germ, wheat germ oil, cottonseed and corn oil, whole grains, and green vegetables. Little vitamin E is found in animal foods.

VITAMIN K is a fat-soluble vitamin which influences the body's production of blood-clotting proteins. Vitamin K is synthesized by bacterial action in the intestines. Sources include green and yellow vegetables and leafy greens, especially cabbage, kale, and spinach. Animal foods and cereals contain little vitamin K.

## To B or Not To B

THE B COMPLEX VITAMINS play essential roles in metabolizing energy from carbohydrates, fats, and proteins, and also help to maintain the proper functioning of the nervous system. As the entire B complex are water-soluble and excesses are excreted in the urine, they should be derived regularly from the diet.

THIAMINE, $B_1$, is a regulator in carbohydrate metabolism. It also helps in the function of the nervous system. Sources include brewer's yeast, wheat germ, legumes (especially peas and soybeans), oranges, whole grains, and enriched cereals. Thiamine is easily destroyed by heat.

RIBOFLAVIN, $B_2$, functions as a coenzyme in energy release; it also helps to activate $B_6$, folic acid, and $B_{12}$. Sources include brewer's yeast, beef liver, and milk, as well as whole grains, almonds, brazil nuts, leafy greens, eggs, and cheese. Riboflavin in solution, such as in milk, is destroyed by exposure to light.

NIACIN, $B_3$, is important as a coenzyme in energy release; it aids in the maintenance of healthy skin, gastrointestinal tissue, and the nervous system. Getting enough protein influences one's niacin intake. The amino acid tryptophan is converted in the body to niacin; the process requires the presence of thiamine, riboflavin, and pyridoxine. Sources include brewer's yeast, legumes, peanut butter, and whole grain breads and cereals.

PYRIDOXINE, $B_6$, plays a major role as part of the enzyme systems that affect protein metabolism. Vitamin $B_6$ also functions in the release of energy from glycogen and in the synthesis of hemoglobin and antibodies. Sources are meats, liver, egg yolks, brewer's yeast, whole grains, bananas, and vegetables.

VITAMIN $B_{12}$ is a crucial vitamin because it interacts with folic acid to govern the production of red blood cells in the bone marrow. A deficiency may result in neurological disturbances and pernicious anemia, symptoms of depression, stiffness, and irritability. Vitamin $B_{12}$ must be acted upon in the intestine by the intrinsic factor, a substance present in gastric secretions. The intrinsic factor binds itself to $B_{12}$ and facilitates its absorption. Sources include animal foods, especially liver. Milk and cheese supply some $B_{12}$, but eggs are as $B_{12}$ potent as a steak.

FOLIC ACID interacts with $B_{12}$ to produce red blood cells, functions with the body's enzyme system, and is especially important when cells are rapidly reproducing or being synthesized. Sources include leaf lettuce, legumes, spinach, oranges, bananas, mushrooms, nuts, and grains.

PANTOTHENIC ACID, like other members of the B complex, functions as part of the body's enzyme system. It is important in the release of energy and in the synthesis of many body compounds. Sources include liver and kidney, as well as nonflesh sources of brewer's yeast, egg yolk, wheat bran, and fresh vegetables, particularly peas, limas, and broccoli.

BIOTIN plays a role in the body's utilization of carbohydrates, fats, and proteins. Sources include egg yolks, milk, brewer's yeast, mung bean sprouts, cooked soybeans, and some fruits, vegetables, and nuts.

The B complex is just that—a matrix of interacting compounds. Get your B complex from natural food sources rather than vitamin pills, if possible. If you decide after reading about vitamin supplements that you want to take a B complex vitamin pill, it should be taken with meals so all nutrients are present at the same time.

### Minerals

MINERALS are necessary to the body as chemical regulators and as construction materials. Calcium, chlorine, magnesium, phosphorus, potassium, sodium, and sulphur are the minerals found in large amounts in the human body. Chromium, cobalt, copper, fluorine, iodine, iron, manganese, molybdenum, selenium, and zinc are found in small amounts, and thus are labeled as trace elements.

CALCIUM makes up about two percent of an adult's body weight, more than any other mineral. Ninety-nine percent of the body calcium is found in the bones and teeth, but it also affects nerve impulses, enzyme activation, blood clotting, and muscular contraction and relaxation. Sources include milk and milk products (yogurt, hard cheeses, cottage cheese), kale, mustard, collards, spinach, chard, beet greens, and rhubarb. Other sources include blackstrap molasses, soybeans, figs, apricots, and dates.

PHOSPHORUS, like calcium, is widely distributed in the body, influences bone and teeth formation, enables energy to be stored and released, and affects all metabolic processes. Calcium and phosphorus ideally should be ingested on a rough 1:1 ratio for optimum calcium utilization and absorption. Excessive phosphorus intake causes decreased calcium absorption in the body. The body then draws its calcium needs from that stored in the bones. Sources include milk, eggs, cereal grains (especially wheat germ, whole grains, and oatmeal), cashews, peanuts, dried beans, and peas. Brewer's yeast is naturally high in phosphorus.

SODIUM, CHLORIDE, and POTASSIUM work together to control the body's fluid balance, acid-alkaline ratio, nerve responses, and muscular contractions. Most Americans eat far more sodium than their bodies require. Heavy use of table salt, prepared foods, snacks, and sodium compound additives (monosodium glutamate, sodium nitrate, sodium citrate) causes the public to ingest anywhere from two to six times more sodium than needed. Added salt, like table sugar, is an acquired taste and habit. Provided one has access to sodium bearing foods, no added salt is necessary in the diet. (Additional salt may be needed in the diets of people doing hard physical labor or large amounts of exercise in extreme heat.) Exercisers who sweat large amounts should possibly consider taking potassium. Sources of potassium include meats, milk, eggs, seafood, seaweed, and table salt. Especially rich sources are brewer's yeast, bran, potatoes, molasses, bananas, and oranges.

MAGNESIUM is found in bones and soft tissues and acts as a catalyst in the release of energy, synthesis of body compounds, absorption and transportation of nutrients, the transmission of nerve impulses, and muscle contractions. (12) Magnesium helps keep the calcium in balance. If the magnesium is low, the calcium will be low. Sources of magnesium include seafood, seaweed, soy flour, nuts, whole grains, molasses, sesame seeds, and fresh green vegetables. (Magnesium is part of the chlorophyll molecule.)

SULPHUR is found in every cell of the body and is related to protein activity. Sources include wheat germ, cheese, peanuts, lentils, kidney beans, lean beef, and clams.

IRON combines with protein to form hemoglobin, the substance that carries oxygen from the lungs to the organs and muscles. Iron deficiency anemia is a common problem throughout the world, affecting those in developed as well as underdeveloped countries. United States men are relatively free of iron deficiencies, but an iron lack is common in United States women (particularly pregnant women), children, and infants. One reason for this is the increasing reliance on iron-poor processed foods. Getting 18 milligrams of iron (the recommended daily amount for women ages 11 to 50) without getting too many calories is not easy. Some nutritionists suggest that women take iron supplements to help meet their daily requirement. Pregnant women need an iron supplement of 30 to 60 milligrams over the normal amount to insure adequate reserves. Natural sources of iron include liver, eggs, leafy greens, potatoes, dried fruits, whole grain breads and cereals, soybeans, pumpkin seeds, and molasses. The presence of vitamin C increases absorption of iron.

IODINE is an important component of thyroxine, the thyroid hormone that regulates key metabolic functions. Iodine deficiency conditions—principally goiter—have been reduced in the United States by the use of iodized salt. Sources include seafood, seaweed, vegetables, legumes, or grains.

ZINC is important in the maintenance of normal taste acuity; growth, particularly sexual maturity; as a component of insulin; and as an influence on the healing of wounds and burns, as well as numerous enzymatic functions. Highly refined or fabricated foods are low in zinc and other trace minerals. Excessive alcohol consumption can also cause one to excrete large amounts of zinc. Sources include meat, eggs, milk, cheese, seaweed, pumpkin seeds, whole grains, legumes, and some brands of brewer's yeast.

## What About Vitamin Pills?

Some vegetarians, nutritionists, and health food advocates argue that taking vitamin pills is unnatural and expensive; we should get all our nutrients only from our food. This is certainly the ideal approach. A daily multiple vitamin pill cannot make up for a faulty diet.

Unfortunately, we do not live in an ideal world. American food production and distribution is highly centralized; so-called fresh fruits and vegetables lose some of their nutrients as they travel long distances to market. Even if you eat only homegrown food, modern environmental factors may inhibit your ability to absorb fully essential nutrients or may increase your need for them. The effects of untested chemicals, pesticidal residues, pollution, and stress are factors which affect vitamin-mineral absorption.

Should you take vitamin and mineral supplements? Used sensibly, nutritional supplements are cheap protection against the ill-understood ravages of modern society. Still, the cornerstone of good nutrition is a sensible diet, not a drawer full of pills and powders. The best health insurance of all seems to be a well-chosen diet from varied sources and a life free of junk foods, table sugar and salt, chemical additives, tobacco, excessive alcohol consumption, stress, and sedentary living.

# CHAPTER 12

## About Those New Diets . . .

Yes, you can lose weight on a low carbohydrate diet. But can you do it without endangering your health?

Recently the Food and Nutrition Council of the American Medical Association branded the latest proper version of low carbohydrate diets, advocated by Dr. Robert Atkins, as "unscientific and dangerous." (35)

### The Dr. Atkins Diet

Dr. Atkins' diet is essentially a low carbohydrate-high protein-high fat diet. (8) Dr. Atkins recommends that carbohydrates be *eliminated entirely* during the first stages of the diet on the theory that if your body takes in no carbohydrates, it will have to burn up fat, which is included in his recommended diet in the form of cheese, butter, meat, and milk. Atkins feels that by eating foods high in fat content, your body becomes efficient in burning fat. Thus your new fat burner will be more easily able to burn up excess fat stored in your body. Most people who eat no carbohydrates find they stay light-headed and often feel as if they are "floating."

Dr. Irwin Stillman suggests a high protein and high intake of water, low carbohydrate diet. (60) Dr. Stillman's diet makes more sense than Dr. Atkins' diet since it does not eliminate carbohydrates completely and cuts down on the amount of fat.

However, such diets can induce extreme fatigue, a tendency to fainting, headache, nausea, and vomiting. (35)

Prolonged use of such diets containing lots of fat, and often large amounts of cholesterol, may cause the blood fat and cholesterol to rise to very high levels, increasing the risk of a heart attack, a stroke, or other problems, such as arteriosclerosis.

At the start of a low carbohydrate diet there is often a sense of excessive fatigue. A big factor in this symptom is the loss of body salt. In the absence of carbohydrates, the kidneys tend to lose salt and, with it, a lot of water. This is one of the major factors in the early dramatic weight loss often noted on such diets. Usually by the third day of severe carbohydrate restriction, individuals feel they don't have enough energy to carry on their daily activities. The loss of water from the blood leads to a tendency to faint. These reactions are similar to those a person may experience upon getting out of bed for the first time after prolonged bed rest. Many of these symptoms resolve quickly when the normal body water and salt is replaced—and with this, the *apparent weight loss is regained.*

One advantage that Atkins claims for his diet is that you lose weight because of all the calories that are lost from the body in the form of ketones. Most of these are lost in the urine and some in the breath. Ketones are incompletely metabolized parts of fats. They are formed in abundance in diabetics who cannot use carbohydrates and must use more fat and protein for energy. *However, the body does not lose a lot of calories in the form of ketones when one is on a low carbohydrate diet.*

Dr. L. L. Lamb, editor of *The Health Letter,* says:

Even people placed on starvation with no calorie intake do not lose a lot of calories as ketones. Starvation also produces ketones because the body must get its energy then from its own body protein and fat. In normal people at the most 20 grams of ketones can be formed in a day and lost in the urine. These combined losses account for less than 100 calories a day, hardly enough to account for any dramatic weight loss. (35)

## Why Do People Lose Weight on the Atkins Diet?

Much of the initial weight loss with high protein-high fat or low carbohydrate diets is a result of water loss and a decrease in the bulk content in the intestines. (66) As stated earlier with the study of Zuti and Golding, further weight loss on these diets is due to loss of muscle and body protein, rather than fat. (69) It takes a deficit of 3,500 calories to eliminate a pound of fat; it takes less than a 700-calorie deficit to eliminate a pound of lean muscle. This is because muscle contains a lot of water and fat contains very little water.

## Is There Something Bad About Carbohydrates?

The idea that carbohydrates are some kind of bad food or poison is without scientific evidence. As discussed earlier, there are two types of carbohydrates: simple and complex. Table sugar, candy, and cake sugar are examples of simple sugars and should be eliminated from our diet. I recommend 60-70 percent of your daily food intake be complex carbohydrates. This will give you a more balanced diet, as well as eliminate the light-headed effect. Fresh fruits, vegetables, and cereals all contain important vitamin and minerals essential to good health. In normal people, complex carbohydrates do not produce low blood sugar—an almost unknown problem in parts of the world where the diet is 80 percent complex carbohydrates. People on these diets are also less prone to heart and vascular disease than in our population, where fat is a major component of diet. Blood glucose, the principal body sugar, is essential to many cell functions, and in the absence of carbohydrates in the diet, the body metabolism must convert various food stores to glucose to keep the level within fairly narrow limits for proper health.

Fruit, vegetables, and cereals have been a part of man's

diet since his earliest beginnings, and because of the natural occurrence of honey, even the concentrated sweets of the carbohydrate group were not unknown to the most primitive man. Thus, it seems safe to presume that man has long used complex carbohydrates, and they often have constituted the main source of man's nutrition.

## Liquid Protein Diet

The liquid protein diet is a recent scheme put upon the American people. Its only possible good point is that protein can be obtained without eating foods that are also high in fat and cholesterol. Many liquid protein drinks, while high in protein, are obtained from animal protein sources such as hair and hoofs.

Whenever you severely restrict carbohydrate intake you mobilize fat; excess rapid mobilization of fat causes serious side effects, including liver damage. Liquid protein diets also may produce low potassium levels in the blood. The chemical imbalance and the loss of salt, water, and other minerals lead to weakness, faintness, and other undesirable side effects.

## Severely Restricted Diets

A concluding point needs to be made about all severely restricted diets. If there is a calorie deficit of too great a magnitude for too long a period of time, the normal functioning of the body will be affected. A severely restricted diet allows definite loss of weight, but some of that weight loss will be muscle tissue. (See Chapter 5.)

People on a low, low calorie diet develop the appearance we might expect: a wasted face and signs of emaciation. Hair has a tendency to grow slowly and even fall out. The dieters feel chilled even on warm days. Cuts and wounds heal slowly. They undergo psychological changes, including withdrawal and reactions we commonly attribute to aging. Sex drive is lowered. Digestive disturbances such as gaseousness and diarrhea are common side effects.

The lesson is that, regardless of the diet fad that is being promoted, if you eat too few calories too long, there will be unhealthy changes in the way your body functions. The key to sensible dieting is learning how to eat properly and using a balanced diet that doesn't cause you to lose weight too fast. The proper-diet, proper-exercise program combination constitutes a plan you can follow for life and stay healthier and happier.

# CHAPTER 13

## Proper Behavior Modification

I am going to share with you a guaranteed way to lose body fat with loss of appetite (eating less calories) and exercising (jogging). I feel so strongly about this guarantee that *I will personally refund to any reader the cost of this book* if you carry this out and it does not work.

Before I give you my guarantee, please allow me to share a few observations about what the Bible has to say about turning our appetites over to the control of God.

### Changing a Habit

Do you remember how you changed some of your habits after accepting Christ as Savior? Most new Christians find it easy to stop swearing but more difficult to stop the abuse of tobacco or alcohol or food.

After accepting Christ most Christians fall into one of three categories concerning their ability to change a habit:

1. *Change without conscious effort.* A good example of this is foul language. Cursing many times is taken from the new Christian's vocabulary.

2. *Change after knowledge.* Many times after a new Christian gets the facts, he or she is able to initiate a change of habit. One example is food. Upon learning that donuts are damaging to health, eggs and toast are substituted for breakfast.

Smoking can also fall into this category. Learning the facts about how smoking is harmful to health may be all the new Christian needs to make him or her stop smoking.

3. *Spiritual warfare*. Some habits become a battlefield, due to our own pride and rebelliousness. After making a decision to *accept* Christ the new Christian must make a commitment to *serve* Christ. After making a commitment to serve Christ, Scripture becomes an instrument to change lives.

Many Christians know that overeating makes them a glutton. And gluttony is a spiritual problem. The Lord wants us to solve our spiritual problems by the work of the Holy Spirit, as evidenced by His fruits.

Abiding is one fruit of the Spirit. God uses the Scriptures to show us how to abide in Him. If we deprive ourselves of sin, such as gluttony, for 23 hours and indulge for one hour, we are not abiding. Abiding with God is a moment to moment commitment.

Could it be wrong to ask a physician or Weight Watchers to help us with our weight problem when the real problem is spiritual? Only God can help a spiritual deficiency. He must fill the spiritual need underneath, and then He will take away our appetite as we abide in Him.

Let me give you an example. Do you still enjoy making mud pies? Why not? The reason is maturity; you have grown up.

"Put on the Lord Jesus Christ, and make no provision for the flesh in regard to its lusts" (Rom. 13:14). Failure should lead to confession, and confession will bring about restoration. This process is called abiding in Christ. Christ *can change* our eating and exercise habits.

### Can I Really Lose My Appetite for Excess Food?

Deuteronomy 21:20 states, "And they shall say to the elders of his city, 'This son of ours is stubborn and rebellious, he will not obey us, he is a glutton and a drunkard.' " Joan Cavanaugh, in her book, *More of Jesus, Less of Me*, makes an interesting observation. Notice that the elders do not say the problem is gluttony or drunkenness; those are only *symptoms* of the real problems of stubbornness and rebelliousness! (14) It is also interesting to note that the drunkard and the glutton are in the same category.

Perhaps our problem with diets in the past has been that we have not obeyed the voice of the Holy Spirit; that we have eaten at the suggestion of the world, the flesh, and the Devil—all of them trying to bring defeat to us through our eating. Perhaps this is why most diets really fail. They do not call us to change our minds, only our actions. Both must be changed.

Have you asked God to change your heart and mind and help you with your diet problems? The more you learn about nutrition, the more you will learn the foods you can eat and the foods you should not eat. An example we have considered previously is white table sugar. When you eliminate sugar from your diet, your taste buds must readjust. It takes about a week. During this period of time many foods appear bitter because your taste buds have been bombarded with sugar for many years. You will be tempted into thinking that food must be sweetened with table sugar. The only way we can overcome the lusts of the flesh is to call on God and the Holy Spirit to be our partner in fighting this battle.

Psalm 55:18 states, "He will redeem my soul in peace from the battle which is against me, for they are many who strive with me." Have you ever asked God to take away your desire for certain junk foods, like candy, ice cream, or pie? Do you have a weakness for a certain food? Do you find that you *must* have a candy bar every day? God can deliver us from junk food diets if only we will call on Him. Only with God's help can we overcome eating the junky foods that contaminate our temples.

Jesus said, "Therefore I say to you, all things for which you pray and ask, believe that you have received them and they shall be granted you" (Mark 11:24). He further promises,

"And whatever you ask in My name, that will I do, that the Father may be glorified in the Son. If you ask Me anything in My name, I will do it" (John 14:13,14). We have the right to ask for help with *anything*, *any problem*, as long as we ask it in the name of Jesus Christ. Hebrews 11:1 states, "Now faith is the assurance of things hoped for, the conviction of things not seen."

What foods do you eat that you know are bad for you? Do you eat them but feel your appetite for them is never satisfied? Are you overweight? Why not claim this promise from this day forward: "I have been healed of obesity and compulsive eating according to 1 Peter 2:24, 'He Himself bore our sins in His body on the cross, that we might die to sin and live to righteousness; for by His wounds you were healed.' " Being overweight and eating compulsively is just as much a sin as swearing, cheating, or lying.

Psalm 19:14 tells us to "Let the words of my mouth and the meditation of my heart be acceptable in Thy sight, O LORD, my rock and my redeemer." Why don't you take a piece of paper right now and list those foods that are bad for your temple. Pray that God will take away your appetite for these harmful foods that are Satan's tools to desecrate your body. Also pray that God will allow you to learn more knowledge about foods so you will know what is best for your temple.

By now you must have surmised that my promise to stand behind sure weight control is coupled with asking the Lord to help with the past diet failure and future diet success.

### An Agreement

In a few pages I will suggest a contract between you and the living God. Sign it for 7, 14, 30, or more days, and renew it as often as you wish. It is divided into three sections. *Part one* deals with the weight at which you would like to be or that weight which has eluded you on previous diets. We know that your body burns up 15 calories per pound of body weight per 24-hour period of time. Simply multiply your desired body weight times 15 to get the amount of calories you are allowed to eat to maintain that weight.

In order to reach the desired weight, the contract suggests you subtract 500 calories per day from your food intake, which means a loss of one pound per week. (Five hundred calories times seven days equals 3,500 calories, or the loss of one pound.) This is a sensible diet which will show a four-pound loss per month.

But wait—there are two more sections to the contract! The *second part* of the contract states that you will write down an exact exercise schedule which you can follow, with the Lord's help, for six days a week, Monday through Saturday. Rest one day per week on Sunday, the Lord's Day. Needless to say, this exercise will contribute greatly to the loss of unwanted pounds of fat.

The *third part* of the contract states that you will covenant to begin and end each day with prayer, asking God specifically for mastery over food and drink, and read a chapter of Proverbs each morning.

## Four Promises for You

The contract also claims four promises of God which you can rely upon as you keep your agreement with God. The Scriptures are an excellent vehicle through which you will be able to lose those ugly pounds of fat, and do it in the power of Christ, not by relying on your own courage and willpower. (I have failed so often when I relied on my own willpower—have you?) You would do well to run this agreement by your pastor as well, both for his nod of approval and for his support as you live it out.

First Corinthians 10:13 states, "No temptation has overtaken you but such as is common to man; and God is faithful, who will not allow you to be tempted beyond what you are able, but with the temptation will provide *the way* of escape also, that you may be able to endure it" (italics mine). Have you ever asked God to help you overcome the temptation of food? Have you ever asked Him to help you learn what foods are high in caloric value and to take away your desire for those foods?

When I signed a contract with God for one month, I used and claimed 1 Corinthians 10:13 against my great desire for ice cream. Ice cream has always been one of my favorite snacks, or at times a complete meal. I have, on occasion, eaten an entire gallon of ice cream just because it tasted good. After I entered into my commitment to God, my desire for ice cream completely left me. I did not even want to taste it, even though it was offered to me several times during my month-long contract. *God can and will remove your desire for certain foods!* I have decided that the only way I can be delivered from ice cream is to believe God for 1 Corinthians 10:13 for the rest of my life. That's really not so bad. My temple can function better without all that unnecessary sugar.

The contract also claims Matthew 26:41, which states: "Keep watching and praying, that you may not enter into temptation; the spirit is willing, but the flesh is weak." Most of us have tried to use our own efforts to resist while on a diet, but to no avail. Why not pray and claim Matthew 26:41 to resist the temptation of those high calorie, empty foods.

Matthew 18:19,20 states, "Again I say to you, that if two of you agree on earth about anything that they may ask, it shall be done for them by My Father who is in heaven. For where two or three have gathered together in My name, there I am in their midst." These verses advise us to get a praying partner for the duration of the contract. Your wife, husband, or close friend will be very happy to support you in prayer. So if you, your spouse, and Jesus Christ together cannot beat your desire for undesirable food, there is no power in prayer.

Satan is always the loser when he competes with Jesus. God has given us spouses and/or close friends to call upon in time of need. Christians are instructed to call upon their brothers and sisters in Christ to pray for certain problems and situations in their life. Eating the wrong foods, especially high calorie foods, is certainly a problem most of us need help to conquer.

Finally, Philippians 4:13 states, "I can do all things through Him who strengthens me." God will help any person keep a contract written with Him. He has promised to strengthen us when we or our prayer partners call upon Him.

I signed the following contract with God for 30 days. My wife also signed it. We prayed together and we prayed separately for God's help and direction. I lost nine pounds in 30 days, from a weight of 153 to 144. God showed me that this contract *will work with His help*.

After you have prayed about signing, ask yourself the question, "Is there any reason why I should not sign the contract?" Other than fear, I cannot think of any reason why someone would not want to seek God's help in how to start on the road to *keeping* healthy.

After signing the contract you will see how much easier it is for you to stay at a certain intake of calories per day. Each day that you enjoy the benefits of the contract, you can claim the promise of having been healed of obesity and compulsive eating according to 1 Peter 2:24.

Second Timothy 1:7 states, "For God has not given us a spirit of timidity, but of power and love and discipline." God wants us to be bold for Him and to discipline our lives in such a way as to keep our temples healthy.

### What If I Fail to Keep the Contract?

If you fail and actually break the contract, admit you have sinned and then ask forgiveness immediately (1 John 1:9).

God will forgive you. But *don't use this as an excuse* to continue overeating or not exercising or obeying the Lord.

Job 23:12 states, "I have treasured the words of His mouth more than my necessary food." Job is saying that the words of God are treasured more by him than the food necessary to keep him alive.

Matthew 6:19–21 states, "Do not lay up for yourselves treasures upon earth, where moth and rust destroy, and where thieves break in and steal. But lay up for yourselves treasures in heaven, where neither moth nor rust destroys, and where thieves do not break in or steal; for *where your treasure is, there will your heart* be also" (italics mine).

Have you made food your treasure? Are you so hung up on eating that you allow Satan to be a thief in your life—allowing him to rust your earthly treasure? In 2 Corinthians 5:10 we are told, "For we must all appear before the judgment seat of Christ, that each *one* may be recompensed for his deeds in the body, according to what he has done, whether good or bad" (italics mine). The Greek word for *body* is *sommo*, and pertains to our physical, not our spiritual bodies. When *you* stand before God at the judgment seat, will your temple be filled with earthly treasures or heavenly treasures? If you constantly are thinking of what to eat at the next meal, perhaps you need to ask God to use the Holy Spirit in your life to take the desire for food out of your heart and replace it with a heavenly treasure.

Matthew 6:24 tells us, "No one can serve two masters; for either he will hate the one and love the other, or he will hold to one and despise the other. *You cannot serve God and mammon*" (italics mine). Is food your master?

Matthew 6:25 says, "For this reason I say to you, *do not be anxious* for your life, as to *what you shall eat*, or what you shall drink; nor for your body, as to what you shall put on. *Is not life more than food*, and the body than clothing?" (italics mine). We Christians who want to serve God or think that we

presently are serving Him need to look at how we approach
the food we eat.

Is food a large part of your daily thinking? God tells us not
to be anxious for food; it is Satan who tells us to think about
food, forget calories, and serve the appetite. God tells us in
Matthew 6:33, "But seek first His kingdom and His righteousness; and all these things shall be added to you."

"All things are lawful for me, but not all things are
profitable. All things are lawful for me, but I will not be
mastered by anything. Food is for the stomach, and the
stomach is for food; but God will do away with both of them.
Yet the body is not for immorality, but for the Lord; and the
Lord is for the body" (1 Cor. 6:12,13). Eating excess food will
not hinder your salvation relationship with God, but your
health will certainly suffer. You can master your food intake
and appetite with Christ's power. The first part of verse 15
states, "Do you not know that your bodies are members of
Christ?" This verse tells us that the things I do with my
hands or stomach directly affect Jesus Christ.

This contract with God will allow the Holy Spirit to repro-
gram our thinking about food. Satan wants us to be anxious
for food. God does not. Only after we have made a commitment to God will He allow the Holy Spirit to help us with our
food problem. When you sign the contract before God, then
you have taken the first step in your commitment. God will
honor that commitment and allow the Holy Spirit to repro-
gram your thinking as to how important food should be in
*your* life. Have you failed before, trying to stay on a diet?
*Why not allow God to help you?* Take the first step now and
sign the contract before God.

## My Contract Before God For A Healthier Temple

I, _____, do agree to the following three parts of this contract, made before the living God on (date) _____. This contract is good for (7) (14) (30 or more) days between myself and the Holy Spirit whom I claim to help me accomplish my goal until the completion date of

_____.

1. I will from this day forward reduce my intake of food by 500 calories per day (one pound per week loss). (Take your present weight × 15 [which equals your basal metabolism rate] − 500 calories = YOUR DIET. Example: 155 lbs. × 15 = 2325 (BMR) − 500 = 1825 calories per day − YOUR DIET.)

I will eat foods that are nourishing and will supply the necessary energy for a healthful temple. I MUST COUNT CALORIES!

2. I will from this day forward (after a physical examination if my health is in question) start a six-day a week exercise program. I will rest on Sundays.

3. I promise the living God to begin and end each day with prayer concerning my resistance to excess food and to read a chapter from Proverbs each morning.

I claim God's strength to overcome all temptation in regard to my diet, exercise, and reading His Word, according to 1 Corinthians 10:13. I also claim Matthew 26:41, knowing that the spirit is willing but the flesh is weak.

My witness (spouse, pastor, or close friend), _____ _____, agrees with me on the promise of Matthew 18:19,20 that God will allow me to keep this contract. My witness also agrees to pray for me daily concerning this contract. I claim Philippians 4:13 for the strength to resist extra calories, to exercise God's temple, and to read His Word, through reliance on Jesus Christ.

_____ (Signature)

_____ (Date)

# CHAPTER 14

## Total Health

The content of this book, if followed as outlined, will make the reader a healthier individual who has gained a new lease on life. A nutritious diet can only be good for us. Proper exercise will revitalize our bodies to feel great.

If you use the principles in this book, *you will become half a person.* You will be healthier, more pleasing in appearance, more vibrant, more fun to be with. But you only will *be half a person* until you make a personal commitment to Jesus Christ.

Two thousand years ago, Jesus Christ took upon Himself our full humanity so that we might be saved. That salvation is both *eternal,* in that we are given heaven instead of hell, and it is *temporal,* in that through Christ we have the power now to live godly lives. Through Jesus Christ, all our sins have been fully paid for that we might know total forgiveness and cleansing.

Jesus said, "I am the way, and the truth, and the life; no one comes to the Father, but through Me" (John 14:6). He also tells us, "Unless one is born again, he cannot see the kingdom of God" (John 3:3).

One day Jesus Christ will return for His church. But you don't get in by being healthy. It is as the Scripture teaches, through the water and the Spirit. If you have never committed yourself to Christ, do so now. Surrender your heart and life to Him, be baptized into the faith, then take your stand with Him in His body, the church.

And I'll see you in your renewed state as we march together into His eternal city!

# Suggested Reading About Food and Nutrition

## Books

1. Airola, Paava. *How to Get Well*. Phoenix: Health Plus Publishers, 1974.
2. Cavanaugh, Joan. *More of Jesus, Less of Me*. Plainfield, N.J.: Logos International, 1973.
3. Cheraskin, E., and Ringsdorf, W. M. *Psychodietetics*. New York: Bantam Books, 1974.
4. Davis, Adelle. *Let's Get Well*. New York: Signet Books, 1972.
5. Ewald, Ellen. *Recipes for a Small Planet*. New York: Ballantine Books, 1973.
6. Ford, Marjorie. *The Deaf Smith Country Cookbook: Natural Foods for Family Kitchens*. New York: Collier Books, 1976.
7. Goldbeck, Nikki and David. *The Supermarket Handbook*. New York: Signet Books, 1973.
8. Hunter, Beatrice. *The Natural Foods Primer*. New York: Simon and Schuster, 1972.
9. Hunter, Francis. *God's Answer to Fat—Lose It*. Hunter Ministries, 1600 Townhurst, Houston, Tex. 77043, 1975.
10. Josephson, Elmer. *God's Key to Health and Happiness*. Old Tappan, N.J.: Fleming H. Revell, 1962.
11. Lappe, F. *Diet for a Small Planet*. New York: Ballantine Books, 1975.
12. Sussman, Vic. *The Vegetarian Alternative*. Emmaus, Penn: Rodale Press, 1978.
13. Yudkin, John. *Sweet and Dangerous*. New York: Bantam Books, 1972.

## Magazines

1. *Nutrition Today*, Nutrition Today Society, 703 Giddings Ave., Annapolis, Md. 21401.

2. *Prevention,* Rodale Press, Inc. 33 East Minor St., Emmaus, Penn., 18049.
3. *The Health Letter,* Communications, Inc., P.O. Box 326, San Antonio, Tex. 78292.

---

# Suggested Reading on Exercise

## Books

1. Bailey, Covert. *Fit or Fat.* P.O. Box 23572, Pleasant Hill, Calif. 94523, 1977.
2. Cooper, Kenneth H. *The Aerobics Way.* New York: M. Evans and Co., Inc., 1977.
3. Cooper, Mildred. *Aerobics for Women.* New York: Bantam Books, 1972.
4. Fixx, James F. *The Complete Book of Running.* New York: Random House, 1977.
5. Glover, Bob, and Shepherd, Jack. *The Runner's Handbook.* New York: The Viking Press, 1978.
6. Lance, Kathryn. *Running for Health and Beauty: A Complete Guide for Women.* New York: The Bobbs-Merrill Co., Inc., 1977.

## Magazines

1. *The Jogger,* National Jogging Association, 2420 K Street, N.W., Washington, D.C. 20037.
2. *Runner's World,* Box 366, Mountain View, Calif. 94042.

# Bibliography

1. Airola, Paava. *How to Get Well*. Phoenix: Health Plus Publishers, 1974.
2. Allen, T. H., "Measurement of Human Body Fat: A Quantitative Method Suited for Use by Aviation Medical Officers," *Aerospace Medicine* 34:907-909, October 1963.
3. American Heart Association, National Center, 7320 Greenville Avenue, Dallas, Tex. 75231.
4. AMA Committee on Exercise and Physical Fitness, "Is Your Patient Fit?" *JAMA* 201:117-118, July 10, 1967.
5. Anderson, Bob. *Stretching*. P.O. Box 2734, Fullerton, Calif. 92633, 1975.
6. Aronow, W. S., "Tobacco and the Heart," *JAMA* 229:1799-1800, September 23, 1974.
7. Astrand, Per-Olaf, and Rodahl, Kaare. *Textbook of Work Physiology*. New York: McGraw-Hill, 1970.
8. Atkins, Dr. R. C. *Diet Revolution*. New York: David McKay, 1972.
9. Bailey, Covert. *Fit or Fat*. P.O. Box 23572, Pleasant Hill, Calif. 94523, 1977.
10. Bassler, T. J., "Marathon Running and Immunity to Heart Disease," *Physician and Sports Medicine* 3:77-80, April 1975.
11. Brynteson, Paul. "Fitness for Life: Aerobics at Oral Roberts University," *Physical Education and Recreation:* 27-39, January 1978.
12. Burch, G. E., "The Importance of Magnesium Deficiency in Cardiovascular Disease," *American Heart Journal* 94:649-657, 1977.
13. Cardio-Metrics, Inc., 295 Madison Avenue, New York, N.Y. 10017.

14. Cavanaugh, Joan. *More of Jesus, Less of Me*. Plainfield, N.J.: Logos International, 1973.
15. Central Ohio Lung Association (American Lung Association Material), 185 South Fifth Street, Columbus, Ohio 43215.
16. Cheraskin, E., and Ringsdorf, W. M. *Psychodietetics*. New York: Bantam Books, Inc., 1974.
17. "Composition of Foods," *Agriculture Handbook No. 8*, Consumer and Food Economics Research Division of Agricultural Research Service. U.S. Government Printing Office, Washington, D.C. 20402.
18. *Consumer Reports*, July 1980, pp. 410-415.
19. Cooper, Kenneth H., *The Aerobic Way*. New York: M. Evans and Co., Inc., 1977.
20. Cooper, Kenneth H. Personal Communications, January 11-13, 1979.
21. Costill, David. "Heat Exhaustion," *Physician and Sports Medicine*, July 1975.
22. Davis, Adelle. *Let's Get Well*. New York: Signet Books, 1972.
23. Ellestad, M. H. et al. "Maximal Treadmill Stress Testing for Cardiovascular Evaluation," *Circulation* 39:517-521, April 1969.
24. Fixx, James F. *The Complete Book of Running*. New York: Random House, 1977.
25. Fox, Edward, and Mathews, Don. *Interval Training*. Philadelphia: W. B. Saunders, 1974.
26. Fox, Dr. Edward L., Personal Communication, Professor of Physical Education, Associate Director, Exercise Physiology Research Laboratory, Ohio State University, Columbus, Ohio.
27. Fredericks, C., *Breast Cancer—A Nutritional Approach*. New York: Grosset and Dunlap, 1977.
28. Gilder, H. et al, "Components of Weight Loss in Obese Patients Subjected to Prolonged Starvation," *Journal of Applied Physiology* 23:304-310, September 1967.
29. Glover, Bob, and Shepherd, Jack. *The Runner's Handbook*. New York: Viking Press, 1978
30. Gly-Oxide Chart—Distributed by Marion Laboratories, Inc., 10236 Bunker Ridge Road, Kansas City, Mo. 64137.

31. Goldman, R., and Buskirk, E. *Body Volume Measurements by Underwater Weighing, Description of a method in techniques for measuring body composition.* Washington, D.C.: National Academy of Science, 1961, pp. 78-89.
32. Greene, G. E. "Non-Smoker's Rights: A Public Health Issue," *JAMA* 239:2125-2127, May 19, 1978.
33. *The Health Letter,* Volume II, Number 8, P.O. Box 326, San Antonio, Tex. 78292.
34. *The Health Letter,* Volume XII, Number 4, P.O. Box 326, San Antonio, Tex. 78292.
35. *The Health Letter,* Volume II, Number 2, P.O. Box 326, San Antonio, Tex. 78292.
36. *The Health Letter,* Volume I, Number 11, P.O. Box 326, San Antonio, Tex. 78292.
37. *The Health Letter,* Volume IX, Number 5, P.O. Box 326, San Antonio, Tex. 78292.
38. *The Health Letter,* Volume IX, Number 8, P.O. Box 326, San Antonio, Tex. 78292.
39. Henderson, Joe. *Run Gently, Run Long.* Mountain View, Calif.: World Publications, 1974.
40. Hickey, W. B. et al. "Study of Coronary Risk Factors Related to Physical Activity in 15,171 Men," *British Medical Journal* 3:507-509, 1975.
41. Higdon, Hal. *Fitness After Forty.* Mountain View, Calif.: World Publications, 1977.
42. Kannell, W. "The Framingham Heart Study Habits and Coronary Heart Disease," *Public Health Service Publication No. 1515,* U.S. Government Printing Office, Washington, D.C., 1966.
43. Kannell, W., and Gordon, T. "An Epidemiological Investigation of Cardiovascular Disease," *Public Health Service,* Section 30, U.S. Government Printing Office, Washington, D.C., 1974.
44. Keys, Ancel. "Calories at Rest," *Metabolism* VII 22, No. 4, April 1973.
45. Lamb, Dr. L. L. *The Health Letter,* Volume II, Number 9, P.O. Box 326, San Antonio, Tex. 78292.
46. Lamb, L. L., Medical Columnist for Newspaper Enterprise Association and formerly Professor of Medicine at Baylor

College of Medicine, P.O. Box 326, San Antonio, Tex. 78292.

47. McGregor, M., "The Coronary Collateral Circulation," *Circulation* 52:529-530, October 1975.

48. Miller, G. J. "Plasma-High-Density-Lipoprotein Concentration and Development of Ischaemic Heart Disease," *Lancet* 1: 16-9, January 4, 1975.

49. "Self Testing and Health Maintenance," *The Jogger*, No. 25, June 1974.

50. Paffenberger, R. S., Jr., and Hale, W. E. "Work Activity and Coronary Heart Mortality," *New England Journal of Medicine* 292:545-550, March 13, 1975.

51. Palmer, R. E. "Will National Health Insurance Improve the Health of the American People?" *Newsweek*, June 6, 1977.

52. Pearce, J. "Cigarettes: Is There a Plot To Keep You Hooked?" *Family Health*, June 1978, pp. 20-23, 54.

53. *Physician and Sports Medicine* 8 (7):15, July 1980.

54. Pollock, M. L. et al. "Physiologic Responses of Men 49-65 Years of Age to Endurance Training," *American Geriatrics Society Journal* 24:97-104, 1976.

55. President's Council on Physical Fitness and Sports, 400 6th Street, S.W., Washington, D.C. 20201.

56. Reuben, David. *The Save Your Life Diet.* New York: Ballantine Books, 1975.

57. *Runner's World Magazine*, World Publications, P.O. Box 366, Mountain View, Calif. 94042.

58. Ryan, A. J. et al. "Charting the Factors of Fatness: A Round Table," *Physician and Sports Medicine* 3 (7):57-70, July 1975.

59. Sheehan, George. *Runner's World Magazine*, World Publications, Box 366, Mountain View, Calif. 94042.

60. Stillman, Irwin. *The Doctor's Quick Weight Loss Diet.* Englewood Cliffs, N.J.: Prentice-Hall, 1967.

61. Sussman, Vic. *The Vegetarian Alternative.* Emmaus, Penn.: Rodale Press, 1978.

62. Thomas, Vaughan. *Science and Sport: How to Measure and Improve Athletic Performance.* Boston: Little, Brown, 1970.

63. Trager, James. *The Belly Book.* New York: Grossman Publications, Inc., 1972.

64. *U.S. News and World Report*, March 5, 1979, pp. 40-41.

65. Wilson, P. K. *Adult Fitness and Cardiac Rehabilitation.* Baltimore: University Park Press, 1975.
66. Worthington, B. S. "Balanced Low-Calorie vs. High-Protein-Low-Carbohydrate Reducing Diets," *Journal of American Dietetic Association*, 64:47-51, January 1974.
67. Yudkin, John. *Sweet and Dangerous.* New York: Bantam Books, 1972.
68. Zusy, Anne. "Non-Smokers' Fresh Air Fight Getting Fiery," *Columbus Dispatch*, August 1978.
69. Zuti, W. B., and Golding, L. A. "Comparing Diet and Exercise as Weight Reduction Tools," *Physician and Sports Medicine* 4: 49-53, January 1976.